EROTIC MASSAGE

BODY MAGIC

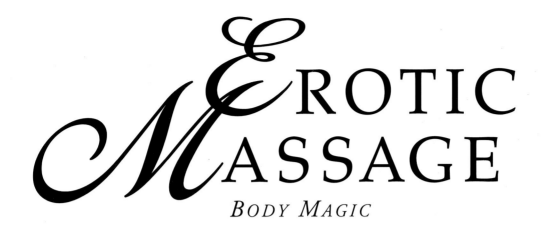

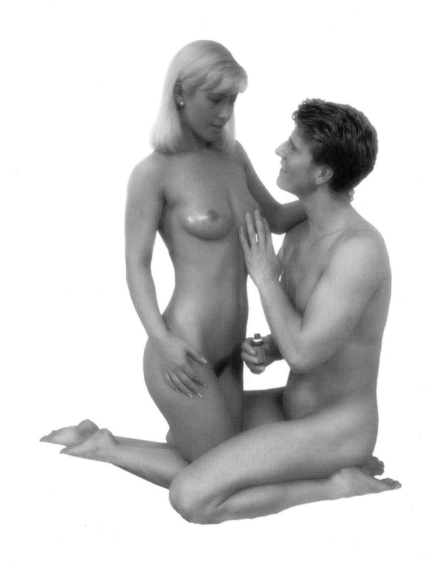

D1292703

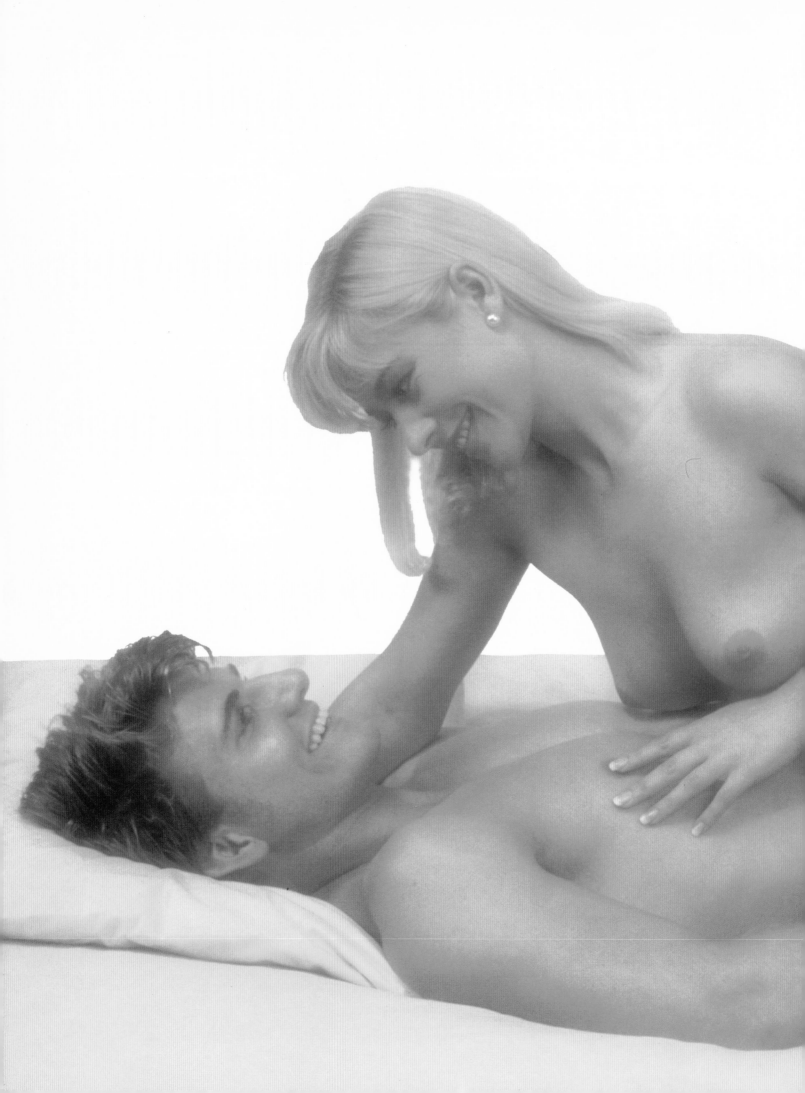

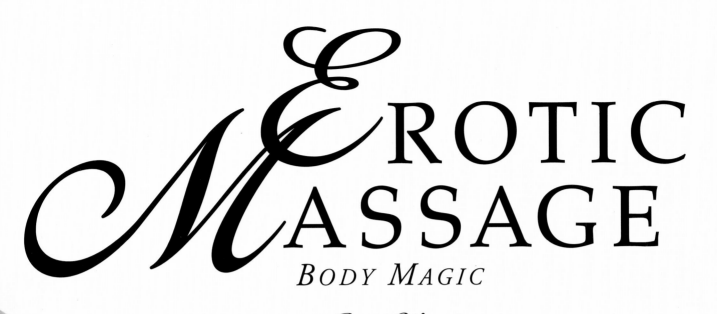

EROTIC MASSAGE

BODY MAGIC

Janet Wright
Photography by Peter Pugh-Cook

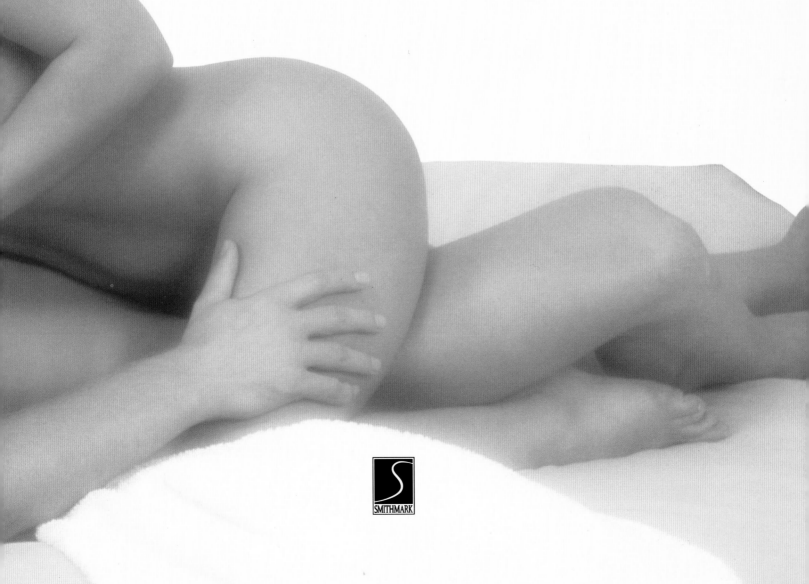

SMITHMARK

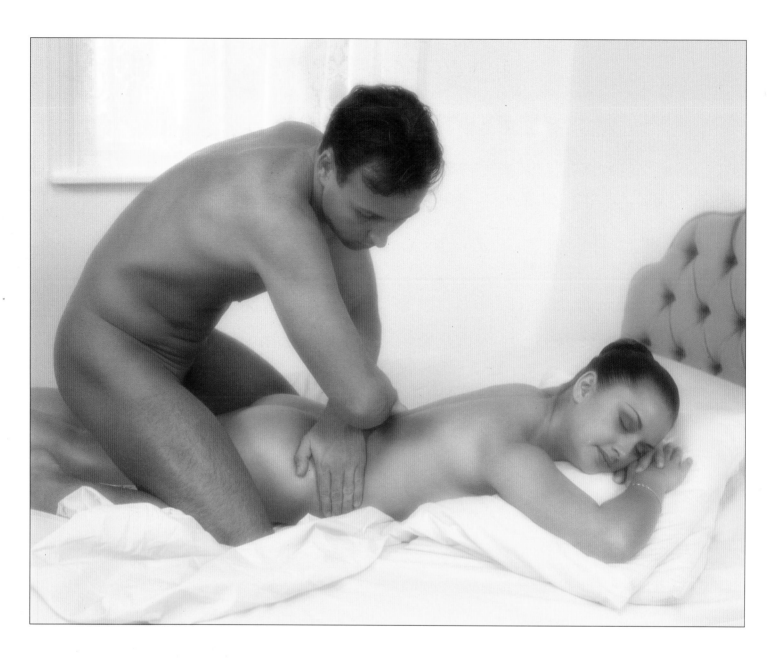

This edition published in 1997 by SMITHMARK
Publishers, a division of
U.S. Media Holdings, Inc.,
16 East 32nd Street,
New York, NY 10016.

SMITHMARK books are available for bulk purchase
for sales promotion and premium use. For details write
or call the manager of special sales, SMITHMARK
Publishers, 16 East 32nd Street, New York, NY 10016;
(212) 532-6600

First published in Great Britain by
Parragon
Units 13-17, Avonbridge Trading Estate,
Atlantic Road, Avonmouth,
Bristol BS11 9QD United Kingdom

Designed, produced and packaged by Touchstone
Old Chapel Studio, Plain Road, Marden, Tonbridge,
Kent TN12 9LS United Kingdom

All pictures © Parragon

ISBN 0-7651-9591-7

Printed in Italy

DISCLAIMER
The positions and advice detailed in this book assumes
that you are a normally healthy adult. Therefore the
author, publishers, their servants or agents cannot
accept responsibility for loss or damage suffered by
individuals as a result of attempting a position or
activity referred to in this book. It is strongly
recommended that individuals suffering from, or with
a history of, high blood pressure, heart disease or any
other medical condition, undertake demanding
physical exertion only after seeking professional advice
from their doctor.

Contents

The Power of Touch

Of all the body's senses, touch is the most intimate. It's a way of communicating without words, at the deepest level. It conveys comfort, love, affection and sympathy. It aids relaxation and healing and is central to our erotic experiences.

The feel of another human body gives more pleasure than practically any other known experience. Odd, though, that since our skin offers so much opportunity for pleasure, even lovers neglect most of it.

Massage takes the natural enjoyment of touch a step further. A therapeutic massage, from a friend or a professional masseur, is a treat in itself – and a revelation to anyone who thought physical pleasure could only be connected with sex. But when you add massage to love-making, it creates a whole different dimension. It brings the entire body to life, extending the pleasure of sex to every inch of our skin.

For most of us, sex happens in a few square inches of the body, with maybe a quick detour to the nipples. With massage, you discover the whole body can be an erogenous zone. Erotic massage is about realising the whole body's potential for sensuous pleasure. It often leads naturally into lovemaking, providing a more satisfying all-over orgasm. But it can be a perfect sexual experience by itself, for a change.

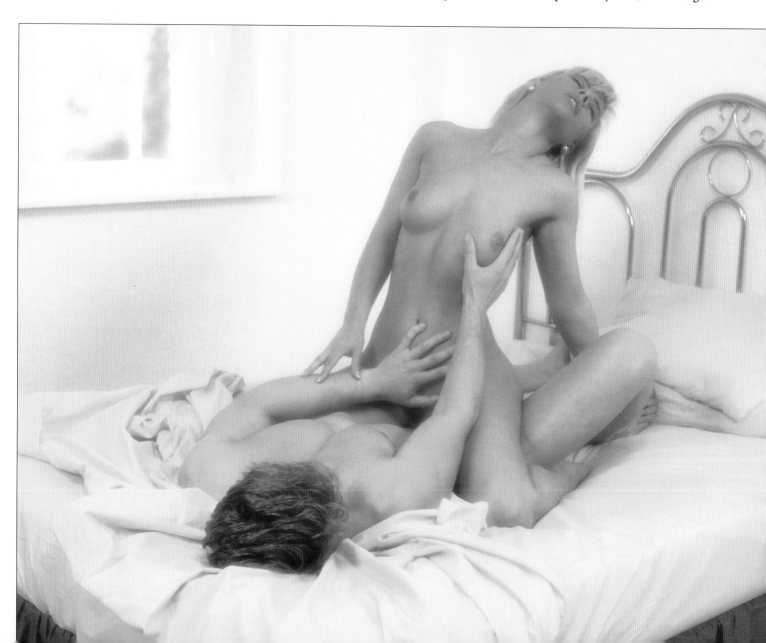

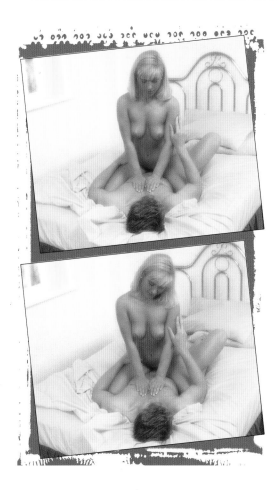

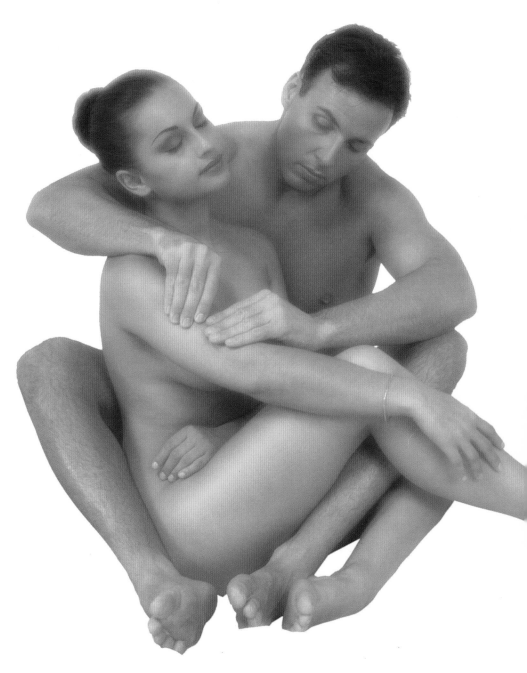

For new lovers, it's a way of getting to know each other's body. Funny how touch is almost more intimate than sex: sleeping with someone may be easy, but holding hands in public is a big statement. Massage bridges the gap between sex and real intimacy.

For others, it's a scenic route to pleasure, offering more diversions than they first think. It can arouse or delay, opening up a world of new sensations. Suddenly your whole body becomes a playground of infinite variations.

If a couple is having sexual problems, massage is the ideal way to share pleasures of the flesh without worrying whether they can have intercourse. It spreads the sexual focus out to include the whole body, and relieves anxiety about 'making it'. As often as not, it leads on to the best climaxes they've ever had.

In these stressful days, people often find themselves too tired or tense to think of sex. Massage is a loving way of helping each other relax – all the better if it leads on to more erotic pursuits. The basic techniques are wonderfully flexible, so different moves can be used to calm or stimulate.

Massage is a path back to pleasure when a relationship is still good but the sex has worn off. Maybe you've been together a long time, or you're exhausted by work and childcare, or you've just got bored with it.

Instead of looking for someone new to get bored with, this is a chance to widen your scope for bodily enjoyment. Revealing a new world of physical sensation, massage creates a subtle and erotic path back to the pleasure you used to share . . . and possibly more than you ever guessed.

If either of you is feeling less lustful than you'd like, massage can arouse desire through a slow, sensuous spreading of pleasure throughout your body. Don't think about whether it will lead to sexual intercourse or not. Just immerse yourself in what you're feeling – whether you're giving or receiving the massage.

Massage for All

Massage has a life of its own outside the erotic repertoire. It has been enjoyed all over the world for its various benefits since civilization began. It's one of the kindest things friends can do for each other, too.

Many of the skills taught in this book can be used outside a seductive setting – it's fairly obvious which ones are for lovers only!

After a tiring day's work, headaches, sore shoulders and tired feet all respond to a gentle massage. People don't even need to undress when you're working on their head,

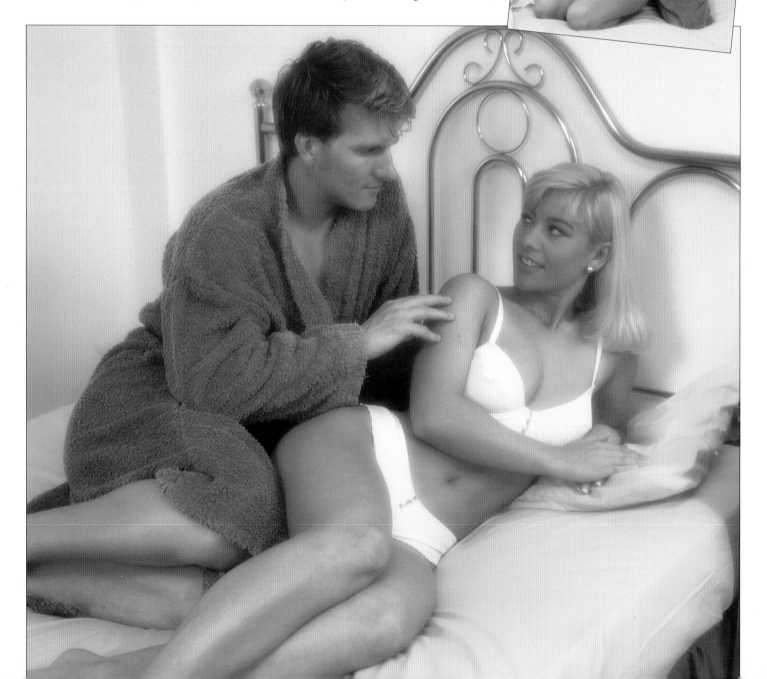

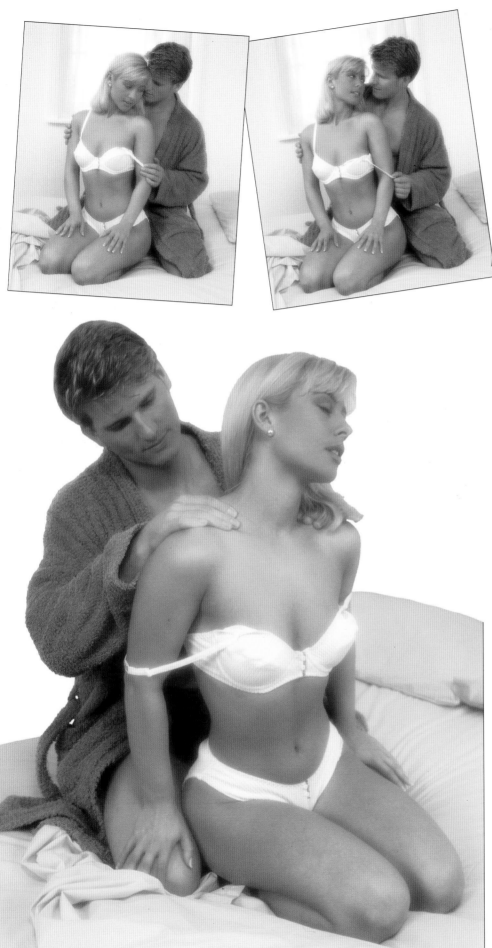

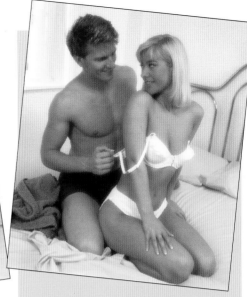

neck and shoulders. Even between lovers, it should always be something to enjoy for itself, whether or not it leads on to sex play.

The skilled fingers of beauticians can smooth 10 years off a tired face, and a good hairdresser will knead the knots out of a tight scalp during the shampoo. Mothers around the world soothe their babies to sleep with a gentle massage. In sports clubs it prevents muscle injuries and in hospitals it improves blood circulation. Physiotherapists work wonders on damaged spines and hungry health-farm clients cheer themselves up with the sheer indulgence of an aromatherapy massage.

As skilled professionals in the healthcare field, trained massage therapists pride themselves on easing the aches and pains most of us put up with.

You don't have to be professionally trained to give an enjoyable basic massage, and you can make it as erotic as you like. Once you've learned some simple techniques, it's all about experimenting with what feels good – and what feels even better.

Relax? That's Not What I Was Planning

What's relaxation got to do with sex? It's probably the last thing on your mind when you're planning a night of fun — you can always relax afterwards. True, really good sex is a great relaxer. But the speedy, stressful way we live can sabotage our sex lives along with our health and happiness.

When we're stressed, our brains produce hormones including adrenalin which speed up our heartbeats and fuel our muscles to run or fight. This was vital for our cave-dwelling ancestors, who often needed to run or battle their way out of danger. But these days stress tends to come from the pressures of modern living.

The stress hormones stay in our bodies, making us ill, and disrupting all non-urgent functions like digesting food or preparing for sex. No wonder stress is the major cause of impotence, as well as many other sexual problems in both men and women.

Tired or hurried, sex just isn't so much fun anyway. Unsatisfactory love-making adds to the stress in your life, leading to

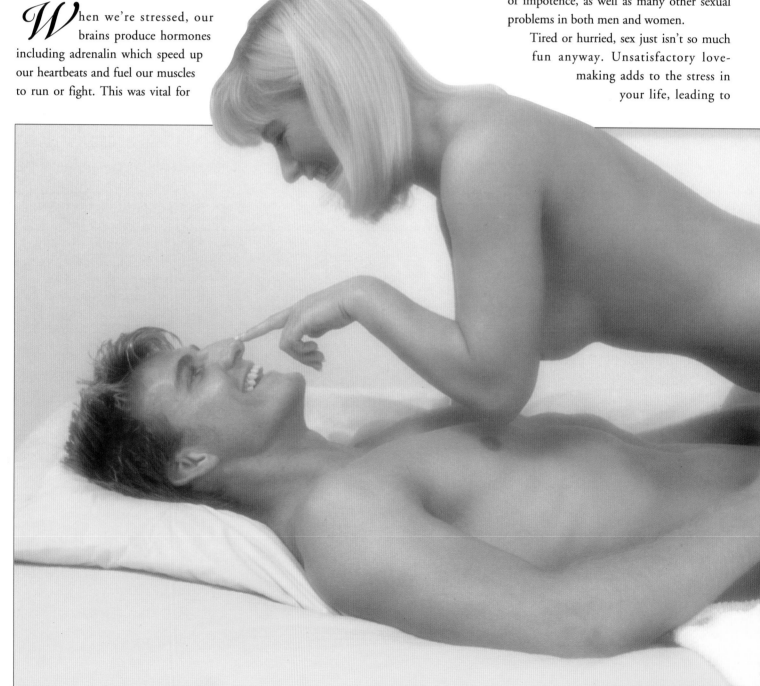

even less enjoyable sex in a downward spiral. Learning to relax (yes, oddly enough it is something we have to learn) reverses the spiral – more relaxed, you have better sex, feel happier about yourself, suffer less stress and relax more easily.

Most of us don't even realize how little we relax. The things we do to wind down – smoking, drinking, watching action films – either disrupt our sleep or cause a physical stress reaction, leaving our muscles knotted and our bodies full of edgy adrenalin.

This is where genuinely relaxing pleasures like massage come in, easing out stress to make room for more enjoyable feelings. And unlike most relaxation techniques, massage can be used to stimulate and excite as well – making it the ideal pastime for lovers.

Start by casting off the stresses of the day, and you can continue with all the imagination at your disposal.

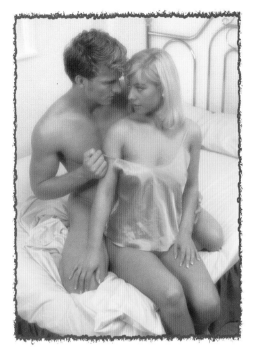

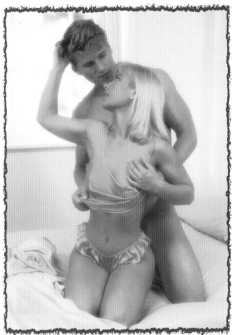

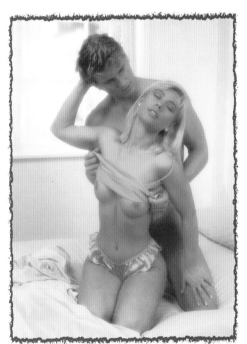

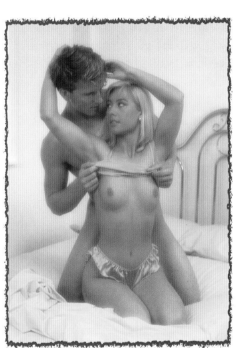

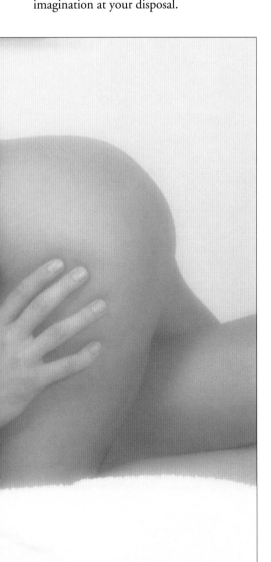

Relaxing with an erotic massage doesn't mean switching off and going to sleep. The muscles are relaxed, but the senses are highly aroused. That's partly because it's tantalizingly slow and sensuous, partly because it awakens the whole body's erotic potential. Easing away the tensions of the outside world, it creates energy for long, slow, world-class sex.

If you don't have half an hour or more to play with, just use one or two techniques, keeping them unhurried – it's the long, slow movements that make massage so sensuous. With sex in mind, this allows a powerful erotic charge to build up. Interspersing some light, fast or teasing movements keeps it moving towards a peak. The longer you can continue, the more explosive the climax will be when it comes.

Shared Pleasure

Giving a massage can be as erotic as receiving one, and you may find yourself changing roles again and again, first rubbing oil into your lover then enjoying the feel as it's rubbed back into you.

Some lovers enjoy sharing a massage, maybe with one working on the other's back and then changing places to receive a foot rub. The most luxurious treat is to have a full-body massage, then lie and enjoy the perfect sensual relaxation without having to reciprocate – but next time you do the same in return.

Erotic massage is something to share. If one partner does most of the work every time they'll soon start feeling resentful and the pleasure diminishes for both. Incidentally, the person being massaged is called 'him' and 'her' interchangeably throughout this book, because massage is delightfully unisex. Women can knead muscles strongly to release tension and men can learn to use their fingers with wicked delicacy. Just give them a chance!

While you're doing a massage, check every now and then that the pressure is right. As you get to know each other's bodies more intimately you'll start being able to feel what needs doing. Your partner too should say if anything is uncomfortable. Most people enjoy massage quietly, but one time to speak up is if anything hurts or you just don't like the feel. Silently putting up with it will spoil the experience for both of you.

The rule in massage is that the person being massaged makes the choices. So if you've offered your lover a back rub, full body massage or whatever but the feel of her body is turning you on, be fair and go on with the massage. It's what she wants most right then. When it's completed you can progress to some seductive moves – and she's more likely to respond enthusiastically.

Listen if she says she doesn't feel comfortable with certain moves or parts of her body, or if you feel her tensing up. Stay with things you both enjoy and, feeling safe, she's likely to become more adventurous with time.

If on the other hand the feel of your lover's hands sliding down your back is driving you wild, tell him he doesn't have to stick to moves in the book . . .

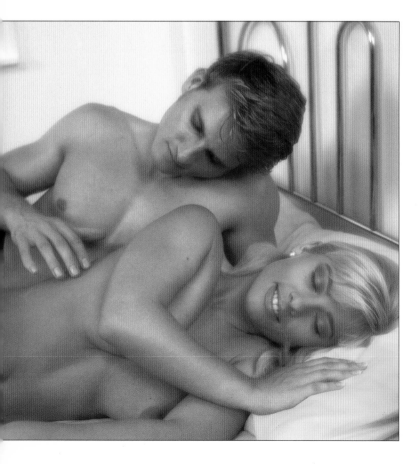
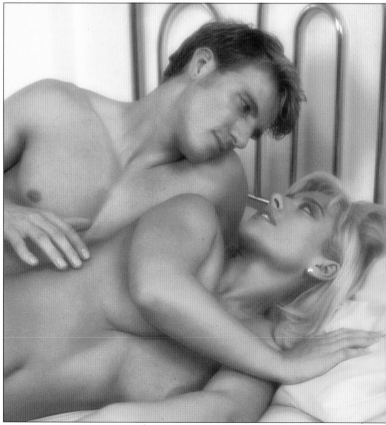

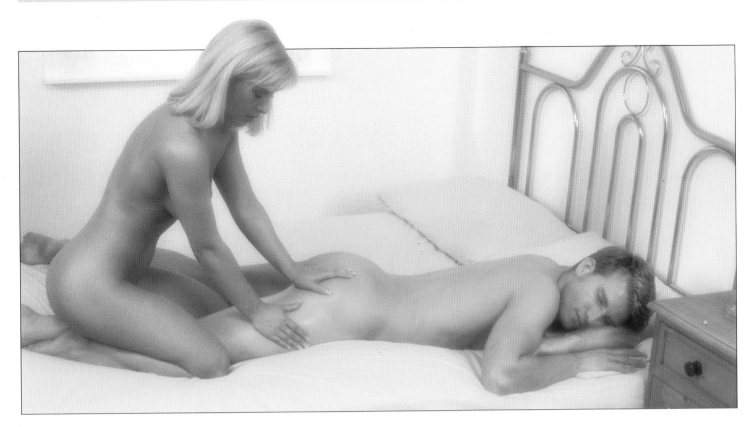

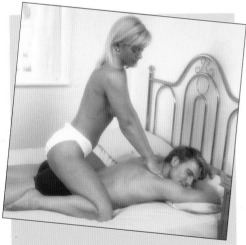

Start a massage by rubbing oil gently over your lover's whole back with your eyes shut, learning the feel of his body and becoming aware of any tightness and sore spots. Take a few moments to work like this on each part of his body as you start to massage it. You'll be surprised how intuitive you can become.

❧

Let the highly sensitive nerve-endings in your fingertips tell you where his muscles are cramped, where he tenses or seems to recoil, where he relaxes easily under your touch and where his body is saying 'More, more'.

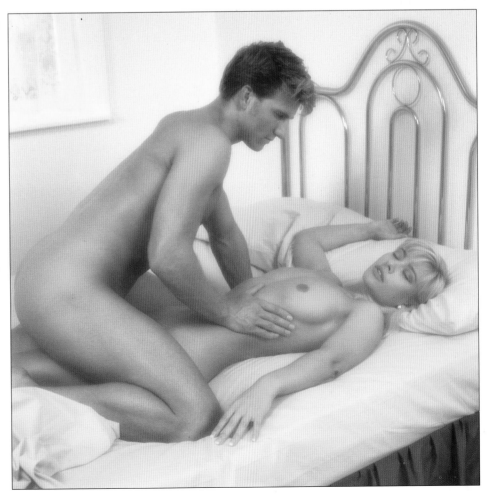

Massage creates a rare chance to become more genuinely intimate with your lover's body and its capacity for discovering the pleasures of the senses.

Not Sure About Massage?

Some men have a great resistance to any touch that isn't sexual. They've been brought up to think their bodies are for work, sex, maybe playing sports – but nothing 'soft'.

Some men often have a horror of things that seem weak or feminine, like emotions for example. A loving touch may even make them want to cry. This sort of man benefits more than most from loosening up, literally, with massage.

He may at first only be able to see it as five minutes' foreplay. But as time goes on he may surrender to real all-body pleasure – a discovery as exciting as his first sexual awakening. Since his muscles are almost certainly knotted with repressed tension, he'll also notice some side-benefits of massage, like easier movement and relief from aching muscles.

Women too may have doubts about massage, especially if they have memories of unwanted sexual contact in the past. Strange though it seems, these bad experiences may leave them able to accept sex (since it's so normal and expected of them) but disliking any other form of bodily contact, and secretly not really enjoying sex that much. Having children can also leave women feeling their bodies are at everyone's disposal and they'd rather be left alone.

If a woman wants to work on either of these problems, massage can be a gentle and sensitive way back to the sensual pleasure that's our birthright. In this case it's best to start with something totally non-threatening, such as massaging her head, shoulders or feet when she's tired. Though even the simplest neck and shoulder rub can help, a real massage using therapeutic techniques like those in this book targets the muscles that ache, in ways that release tension more effectively. She may be amazed at how good it feels and want to explore further. As tension melts away, sex becomes a whole new and rewarding game.

If you want to try massage but your partner isn't that interested, make him a drink at the end of an exhausting day and win him over with a neck and shoulder rub.
See techniques on page 93.

Smooth in body lotion for him after a bath with long, slow strokes up his arms and back. Take time with his feet – the most neglected erogenous zone.

Below: A loving touch could encourage him to be a little more adventurous.

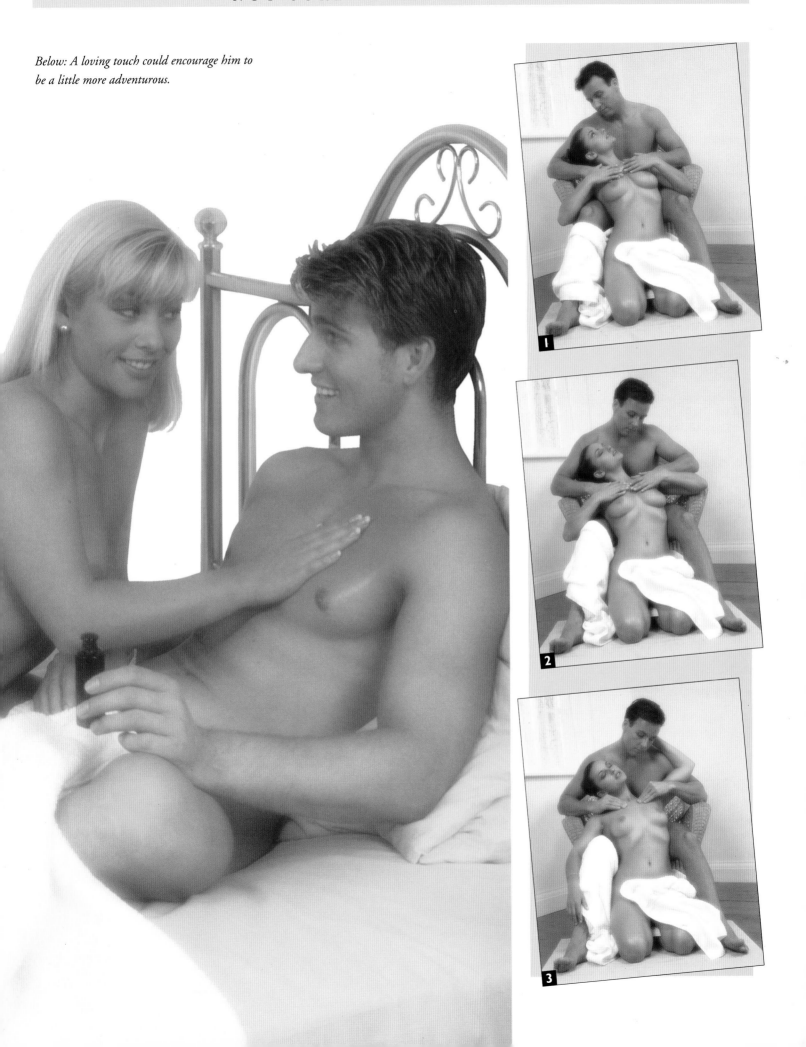

Voyage of Discovery

Our skin has so much potential for pleasure that most of us never realize. Yet taking time to discover and revel in this can bring your whole body to life, revealing erogenous zones you'd never thought of.

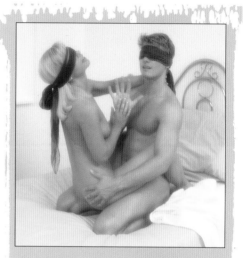

After a bath, kneel facing each other and run your fingers very lightly around each other's faces, heads, neck and arms. Take your time, noticing what feels good to your own skin and how your partner's body seems to react to your touch. After a few minutes, continue to each other's chest, sides and stomach. Next, run your fingers over your lover's legs – avoiding the genital area for the moment, as you're focusing on sensual pleasure in other parts. With arms around each other, rest your faces together and run your fingers over each other's backs and buttocks. You're starting to discover your whole body's potential for pleasure.

Though we evolved with five useful senses, sight and hearing are the only two we use much these days. These are so dominant that they distract

us even when we're trying to use the others. So, when you want to go further, blindfold each other and put in ear plugs to cut out all distractions. You may be amazed how much this intensifies the feeling, in your skin and to your own exploring fingers. Notice the texture of your lover's skin, its warmth and slight musky scent after a bath, the salty tang of fresh sweat, the rasp of hair.

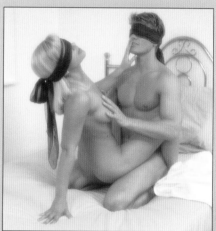

You can vary the routes on this voyage of discovery. Stroke, knead, lightly run your fingernails backwards or forwards, travel with your tongue. Try some of the moves described further on, such as 'dream touch' or 'picking up feathers'. Sit with legs round each other's waists and explore each other with your skin, keeping as much of your bodies in contact as possible as you move.

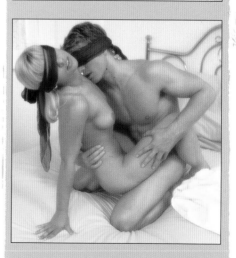

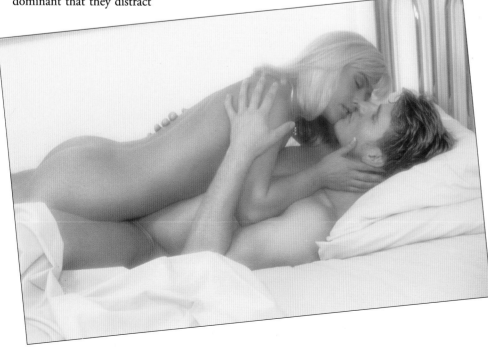

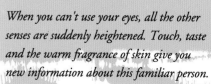

When you can't use your eyes, all the other senses are suddenly heightened. Touch, taste and the warm fragrance of skin give you new information about this familiar person.

If you liked the taste of your lover's body or the feel of their tongue, try adding some other ingredients: cream, wine, honey — anything you'd enjoy licking off each other.

A trickle of cold wine adds a shivery thrill, especially as your lover's tongue chases it down, catching it just before it stings your most tender places.

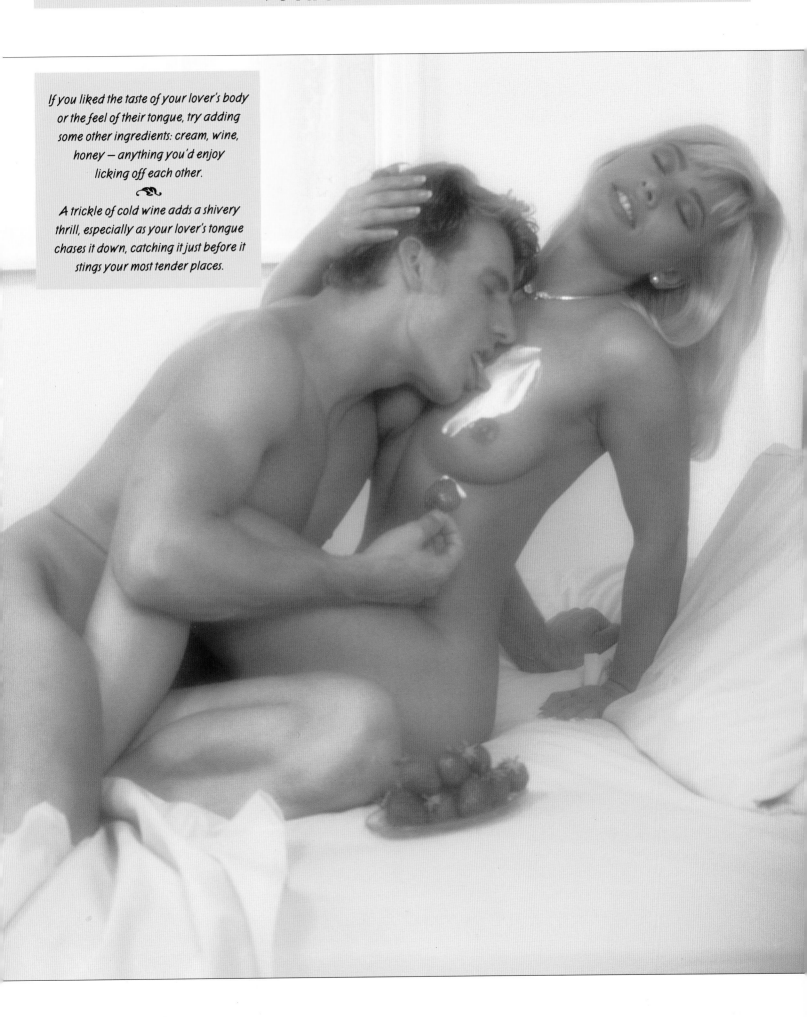

Breathing Together

It sometimes takes a while to wind down enough to enjoy massage after a busy day. Being massaged when they're feeling tense makes some people ticklish, so they tense up even more to try to counteract it. Others become over-sensitive, so that even gentle kneading feels painful.

If you find this, try starting with a simple relaxation technique. One of the easiest and most effective is 'full breathing', which actually triggers the brain to produce stress-relieving hormones. Put one hand on your chest and the other on your navel. Stress makes us breathe shallowly into the upper chest, which triggers the brain to produce adrenalin, which produces more stress.

If your upper hand moves more than the lower one as you breathe, it means you're breathing shallowly. So try to keep the upper hand still and make the lower hand rise with your breathing instead.

It may feel stilted at first, as you deliberately push your tummy out with every in-breath. But eventually you'll feel

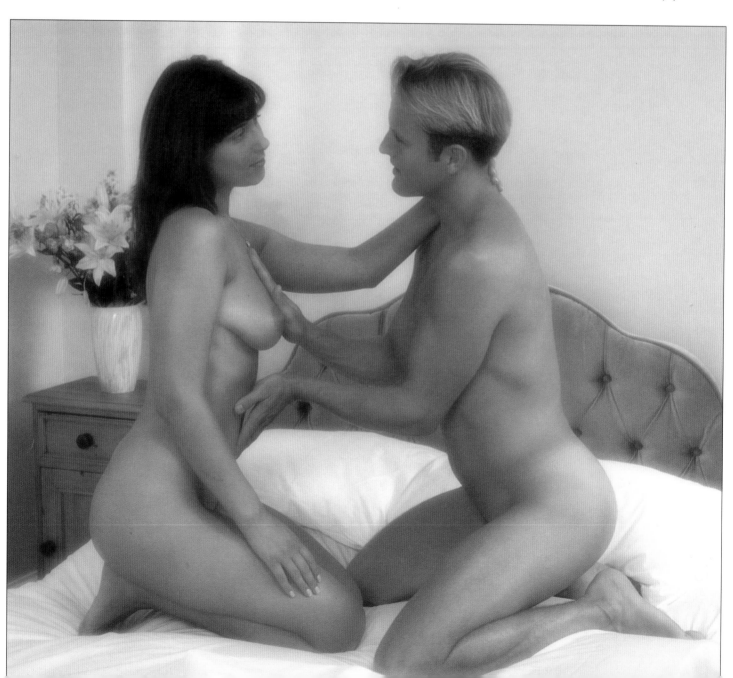

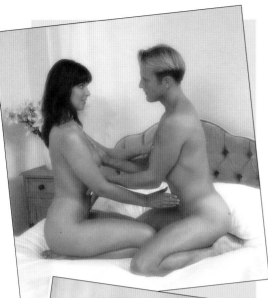

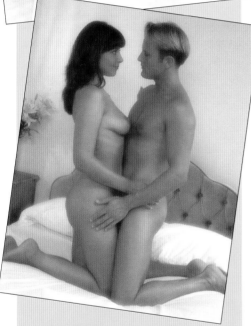

yourself breathing more calmly and fully. Continue for a minute or two, trying to breathe in a comfortable rhythm, not too deeply or slowly. Breathing too deeply can make you dizzy, so stop if this happens and breathe normally. You're aiming to breathe fully, using all your lungs, rather than very deeply or slowly. You can do this exercise any time, anywhere, especially if you feel stressed – putting hands on your chest and navel is just to check if you're doing it right.

A good breathing technique also helps when you need to put some strength into a movement. Breathe in fully, then breathe out as you make the effort. To add pressure, for example, breathe in as you settle your hands in the right place, then breathe out as you lean on them.

Before massage, try the breathing exercise on these pages, kneeling face to face with your partner. Put your hands on each other's chest and abdomen, till you feel the breath entering more deeply than before. Feel yourselves coming more into tune with each other.

Then continue with hands on each other's thighs, feeling your belly press against your lover's as you breathe in. You may start breathing in time with each other, which adds to the feeling of attunement.

Try to continue this relaxed, fully breathing rhythm as you give and receive the massage.

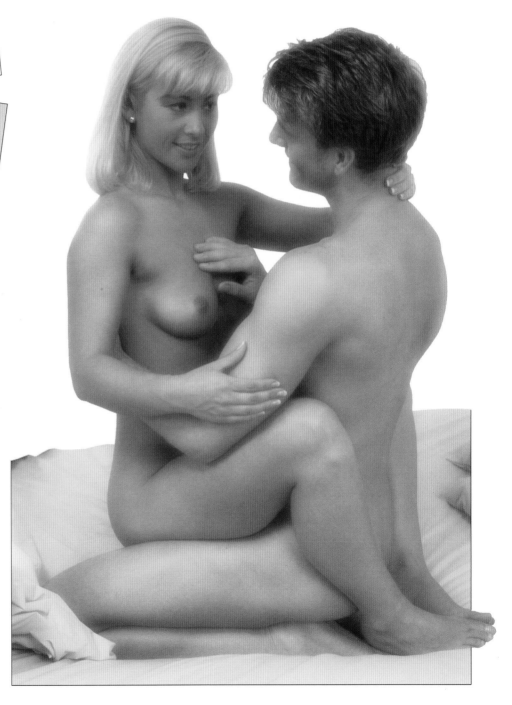

Learning to breathe fully is the first step towards letting go of daily stress. And who better to learn with than someone who's going to share relaxing pleasures with you?

Setting the Scene

Massage is slow and sensual. It can be exciting, relaxing, invigorating, calming, erotic, but it can't be rushed. Enjoying a massage is about surrendering to the pleasure of the senses, and that includes allowing yourself as much time as you can.

You can enjoy massage at any time – a brief neck rub when you're both busy, as a reminder of pleasures to come; some long strokes when you're making love. But the ideal setting to explore all its possibilities is an evening reserved for pleasure.

Start by setting the scene for unhurried enjoyment. A red lightbulb or a coloured scarf over the bedside

Unplug the phone, let the world go away. Tonight you're taking time for yourselves and nothing is going to hurry you.

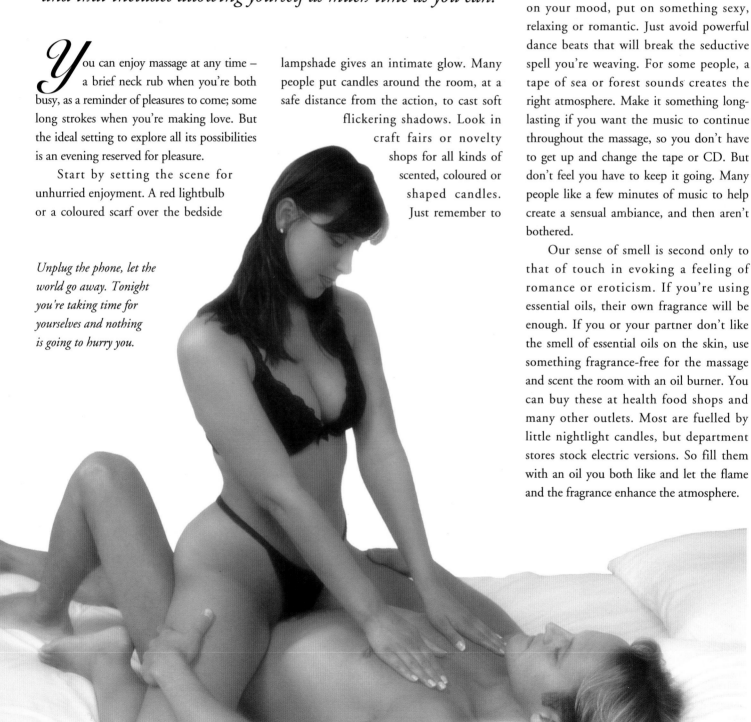

lampshade gives an intimate glow. Many people put candles around the room, at a safe distance from the action, to cast soft flickering shadows. Look in craft fairs or novelty shops for all kinds of scented, coloured or shaped candles. Just remember to

blow them out before you drift off to sleep! For an Arabian Nights ambiance, you can drape coloured cloths or scarves around and scatter some big cushions on the floor.

Soft lights, sweet music . . . depending on your mood, put on something sexy, relaxing or romantic. Just avoid powerful dance beats that will break the seductive spell you're weaving. For some people, a tape of sea or forest sounds creates the right atmosphere. Make it something long-lasting if you want the music to continue throughout the massage, so you don't have to get up and change the tape or CD. But don't feel you have to keep it going. Many people like a few minutes of music to help create a sensual ambiance, and then aren't bothered.

Our sense of smell is second only to that of touch in evoking a feeling of romance or eroticism. If you're using essential oils, their own fragrance will be enough. If you or your partner don't like the smell of essential oils on the skin, use something fragrance-free for the massage and scent the room with an oil burner. You can buy these at health food shops and many other outlets. Most are fuelled by little nightlight candles, but department stores stock electric versions. So fill them with an oil you both like and let the flame and the fragrance enhance the atmosphere.

Undressing is all part of setting the scene for an erotic experience.

You may feel like starting by tantalising your lover with a striptease, hinting at the pleasures to come as you run your hands over your own body.

Arousing your own senses is the beginning of creating a sensual experience for both of you.

Or you can help each other undress, both at the same time, the only rule being you mustn't help with your own fastenings — though you can offer all the encouragement you like.

Too easy? Try undressing each other without using your hands. Now that takes imagination.

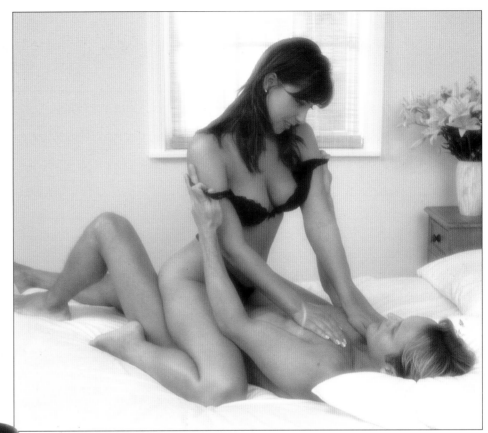

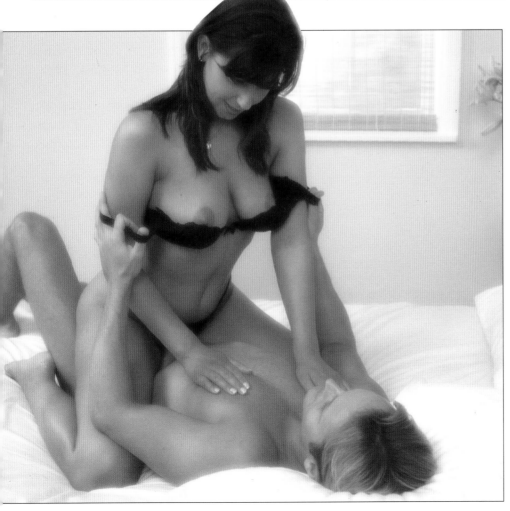

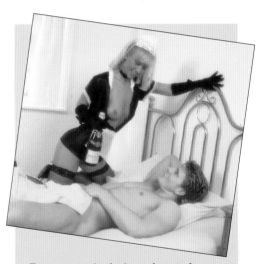

To continue the feeling of erotic fantasy, you could dress up to match.

A woman can drape herself in an exotic silk scarf that she can trail across her lover's skin, or a maid's lacy apron with slightly scratchy edges for a different skin-feel.

If her fantasy takes her to a tropical beach, he can create the scene with a cassette or CD of sea sounds, the smell of sun tan oil and a pair of beach shorts!

Lie Back & Enjoy It

It's important to feel perfectly comfortable when you're being massaged, so you can let go of the workaday tension we all hold trapped in our muscles, that makes relaxation difficult, and sex unsatisfying.

Make sure your bed is not too soft to massage on, or your partner will sink away from your fingers. A futon may be firm enough, otherwise the floor is ideal. An opulent rug to lie on helps create a pampered feeling.

Leave yourself enough room to manoeuvre, as you'll need to move from one side of your partner to the other and from their head to their feet.

Spread a big, fluffy towel on the bed or rug so you won't be dealing with oil stains the next day, and have another one at hand to cover your partner's legs or back when they're not being massaged. A blanket can feel even better if you like the feeling of being pampered and cocooned.

When you're ready to start, just lie down and let the day's stresses drain away.

While you are sorting out towels, add a couple to use as cushions where needed. Some people like one to support their knees when lying on their back, so you can work on their legs without putting uncomfortable pressure on their knees.

Women sometimes like a rolled-up towel under their chests, when lying face down, so their breasts don't feel squashed, especially when you're pressing down on their backs. A smaller towel can be rolled up to use as a forehead-rest when you lie face down; you can lie facing to one side but this may leave your neck feeling twisted, especially when your partner is massaging this area.

Turn up the heating and enjoy the touch of warmth on your naked body.

With your eyes closed you'll feel you are lying on a tropical shore shaded by palm fronds, your body melting under your lover's fingers.

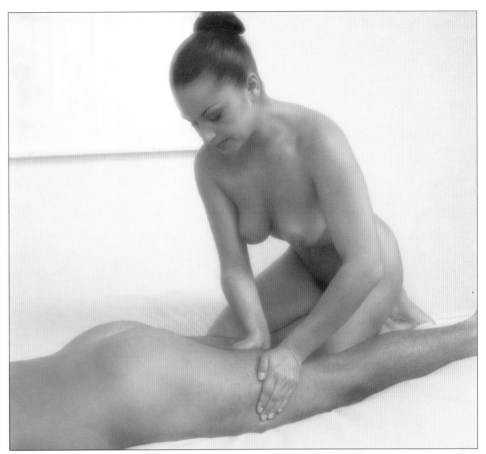

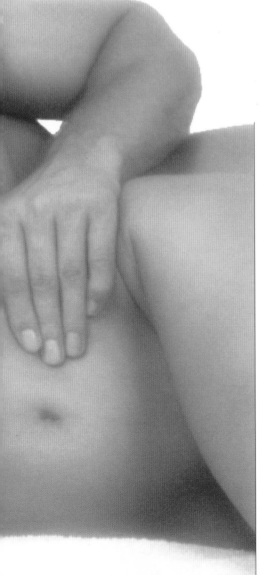

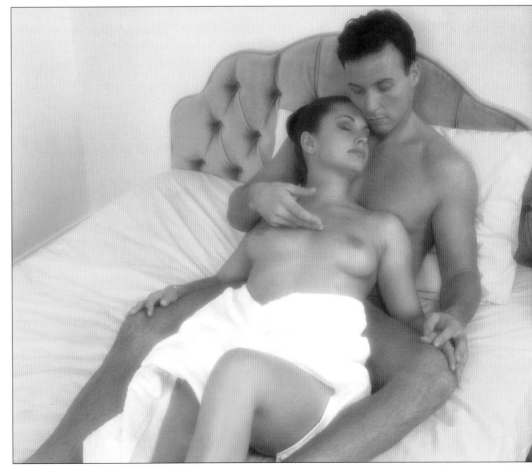

Oils for Massage

Even before you learn any massage techniques, just having oil rubbed sensually into your skin feels pretty good.

Oil also makes massage more comfortable because it lets fingers glide over the skin without dragging it. The small amount of oil used is mainly absorbed by the skin and you can wipe off any excess on the towel when you've finished – unless of course you rub it off on your partner . . .

Aromatherapy – the use of essential oils – is an important part of massage. There's a vast range of different oils, all said to be good for different things. Some are meant to wake you up, others to lift your spirits when you're feeling low, others again to make you sleepy or mentally alert or relaxed. It all sounds a bit weird, but surprisingly, some of these claims have been backed by scientific tests. Which makes things like patchouli, cardamom and rose all the more interesting: they're said to be aphrodisiacs.

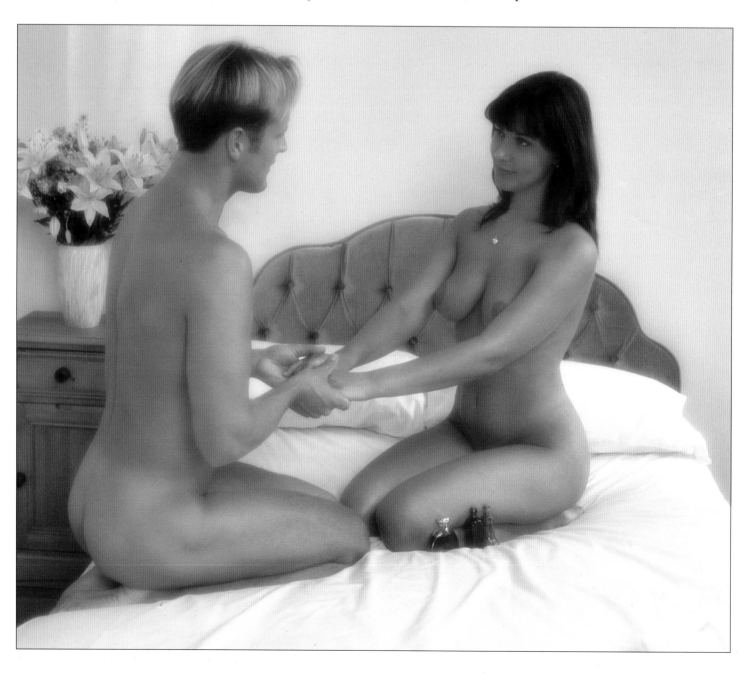

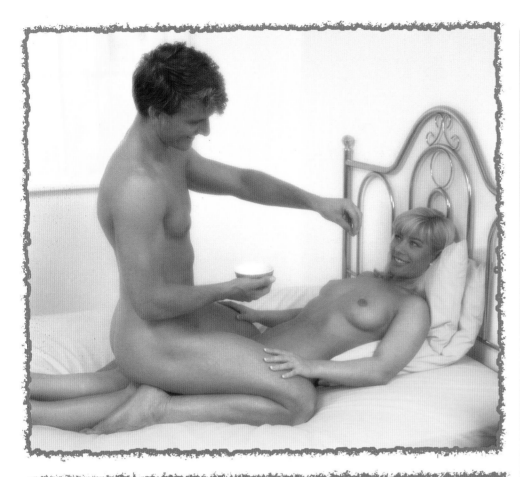

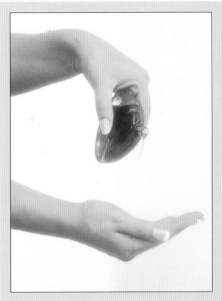

To get used to the feeling of massage oil, choose one with a smell you both like. Pour a little into your hands and breathe in the fragrance.

Rub it into your palms and then into your face. Rub some onto your lover's hands and let him or her do the same.

Stroke it into each other's faces and necks, avoiding the area round the eyes. Rub some onto your lover's chest and smooth it in with your own body.

Gently stroke each other from head to foot. Play games with it: try to oil each other all over without lifting your hands — you'll soon be tangled together. Or spread it all over using anything other than your hands.

These body-games can bring all your senses to life. See where your skin drinks the oil in greedily and where you need very little. Enjoy the smell of the oil mixed with your own natural body scents.

Close your eyes and discover your lover's body with your hands or with your own body, learning it by touch as you glide against each other.

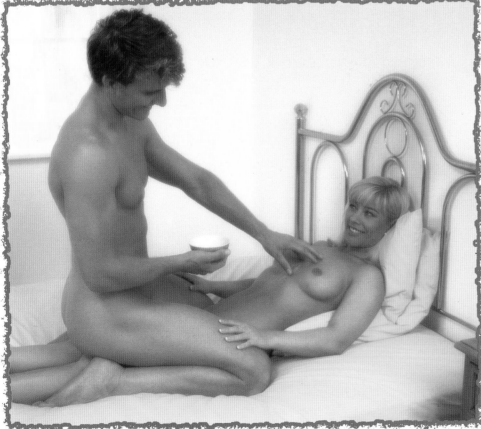

Pour a little of the blended oil into your hands and smooth them together, so that the oil glides onto your lover's skin at body heat.

Essential Oils

These natural, extracts are the concentrated essences of particular plants or flowers that are said to have a beneficial effect on the body. Once added to a suitable 'carrier' oil, they are easily absorbed into the skin, promoting a feeling of well-being, whilst leaving a wonderful fragrance.

Essential oils should be blended with a suitable carrier oil before use, because some are strong enough to irritate the skin. Just add a couple of drops to a 5ml teaspoon of vegetable oil. (If you're using more than one essential oil, use a smaller amount of each – a rough guide is about three drops to a teaspoonful of carrier oil.) Grapeseed is a popular light and neutral-smelling carrier, but don't be put off if you haven't been shopping: any vegetable oil will do in a pinch. Extra-virgin olive oil is even used as a treatment for sore skin or aching joints in itself. Later you can experiment with other textures and scents like almond, avocado, soya, wheatgerm or jojoba. Mineral oils (including baby oil) aren't so good for the skin.

A small amount goes a long way and you don't want to finish up feeling like an oil slick. The amount you need depends not only on body size but on skin type. A dry skin can soak up a lot more oil – incidentally doing it some good. If you make up a blend of about 80mls (16 teaspoonfuls) of base oil, plus 40–60 drops of essential oil, that should be plenty for a full-body massage for two people. You'll soon work out the right amount for you and your lover, and whatever is left over you can put in a screwtop bottle to use later.

True essential oils cost more than ready-blended substitutes, but you only use a few drops at a time. If you're not sure whether an oil sold as 'essential' is genuine and unblended, tilt the bottle to see how thick it is, have a sniff or drip some onto a piece of paper. Most essential oils tend to be rather thin, smell strong and evaporate quickly. Always keep them in dark glass containers, away from heat and sunlight, with their caps screwed on tightly. Once you've blended oils, it's best to use the leftovers within a couple of weeks.

Use the evocative power of smell to excite your partner with a hint of the forbidden: sex in a public place.

If the two of you have a favourite oil or blend for erotic massage, secretly use some of this instead of scent or aftershave when you go out together.

As your partner suddenly recognises the smell, it'll be an intimate message about pleasures to come.

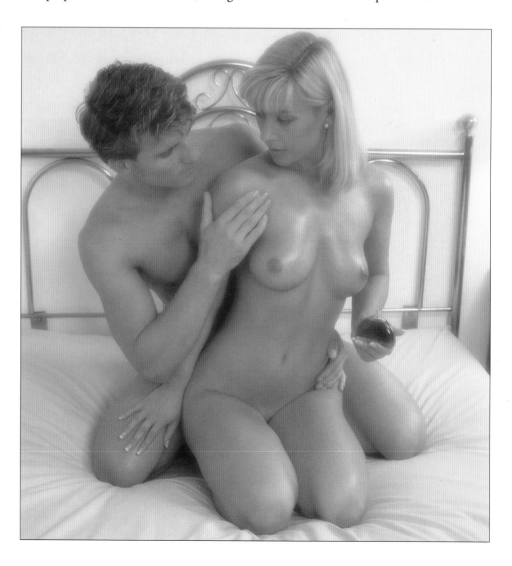

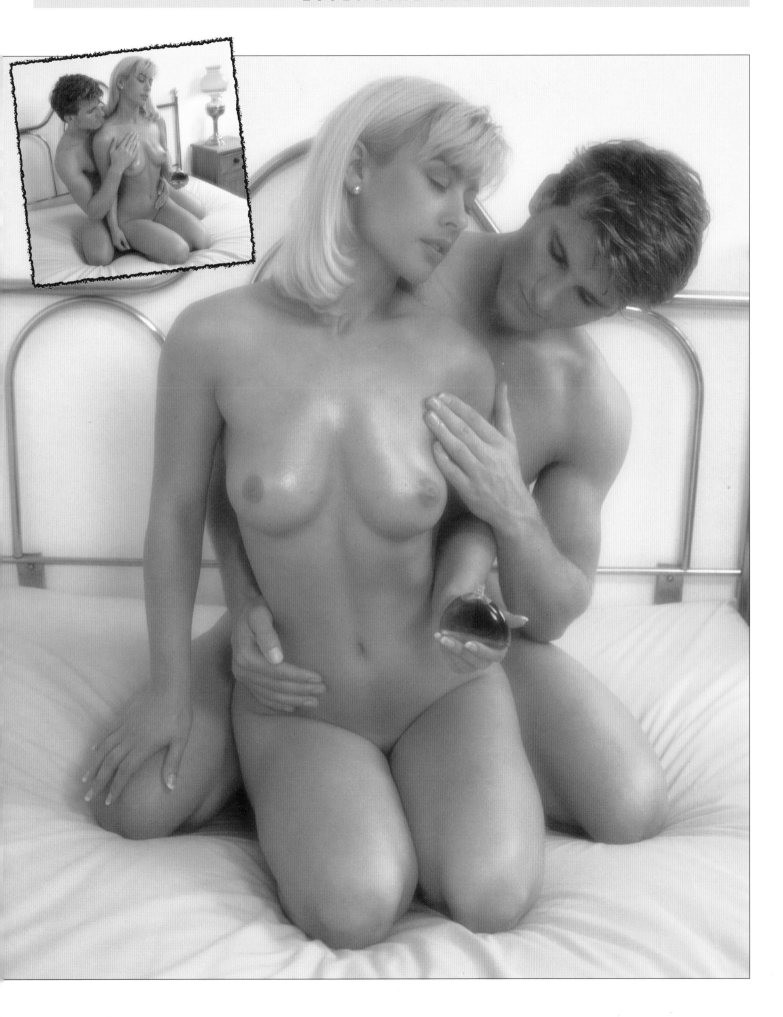

Aphrodisiac Oils

Since time began, certain scents have been known to arouse the senses. Even buying them is a sensuous experience as you share the fragrances with your lover, thinking how it will feel as the two of you rub it into each other's warm skin.

Do try before you buy rather than going by names or descriptions alone. Just as one person loves strawberries while another can't stand them, our reactions to smells are totally individual.

What seems sweet to one person is sickly to another. What you call exotic may smell pungent to me. Smells carry powerful associations too. An oil which is described as

'aphrodisiac' won't do anything for you if it reminds you of something you do not like. So sniff all the testers and go for ones you both like. If possible try them on your own and your lover's skin to see if the scent changes.

Men often prefer the woody scents like sandalwood and cedarwood, while rose is a traditional female favourite. But why not be a bit adventurous? To some people the sweet, heavy scent of ylang ylang is sex in a bottle.

Patchouli is redolent of the mysterious Middle East – great for harem fantasies.

Savour the subtly changing scent as the oil blends into your skin and your lover's.

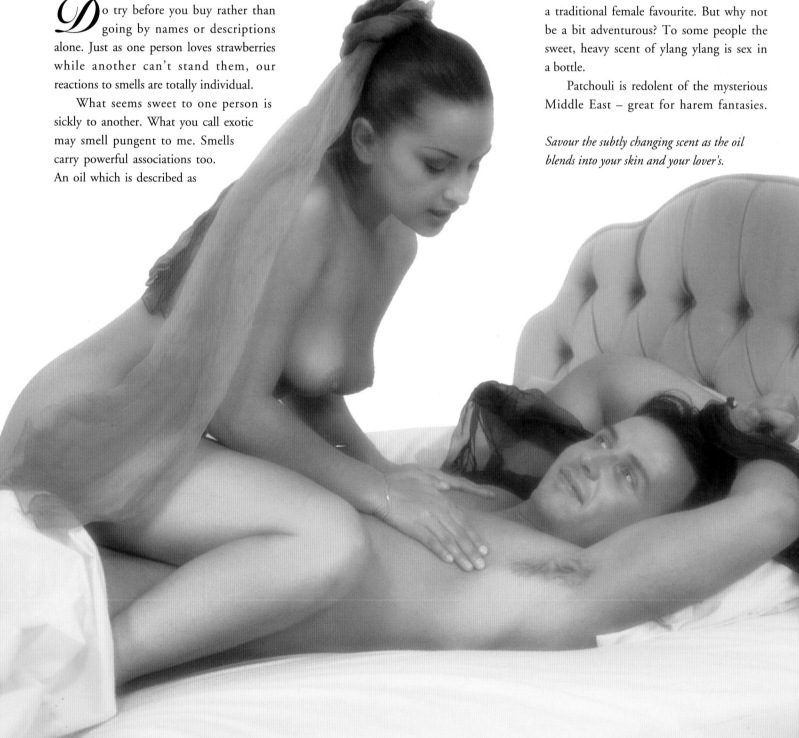

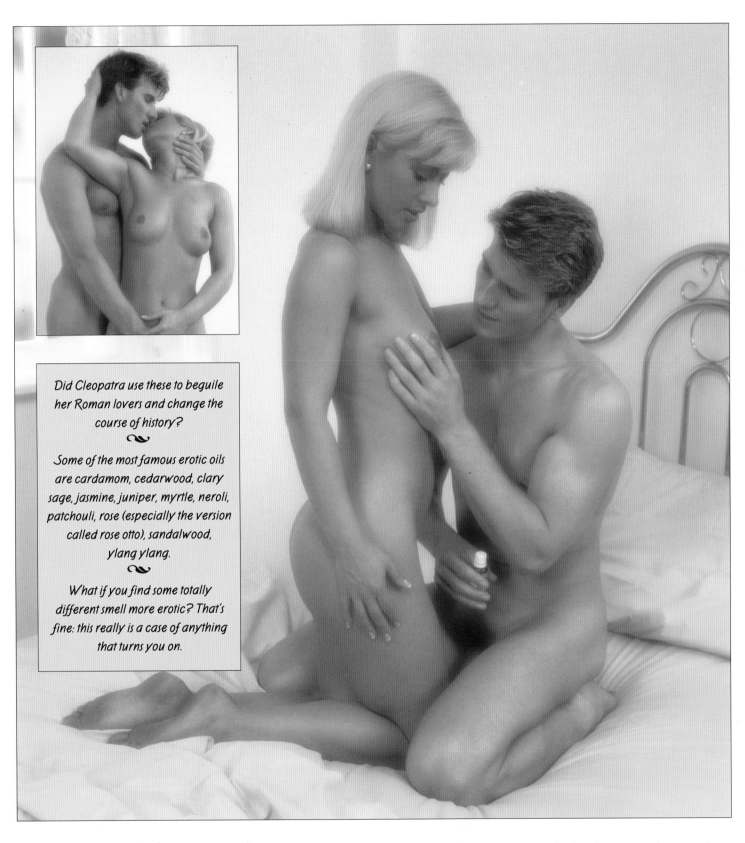

Did Cleopatra use these to beguile
her Roman lovers and change the
course of history?

❧

Some of the most famous erotic oils
are cardamom, cedarwood, clary
sage, jasmine, juniper, myrtle, neroli,
patchouli, rose (especially the version
called rose otto), sandalwood,
ylang ylang.

❧

What if you find some totally
different smell more erotic? That's
fine: this really is a case of anything
that turns you on.

Splash some on yourself and start with a striptease 'Dance of the Seven Veils', letting your chiffon scarves stroke his skin before you discard them.

You can make up your own blends, too. Some of them you'll discover by chance, when one of you, glistening with a favourite flower oil, rubs something with a sharp or woody fragrance into the other.

It starts on your hands but as you both join in the oil spreads all over both your bodies. Legs, arms, bellies press together in a slither of oil and instinct takes over from techniques. Massage soon becomes playing, wriggling, wrestling, love-making. Soon you're rolling together on the floor in a passionate embrace and as for those blended oils – hey, that smells *good*.

Sensuous Alternatives

When you're choosing oils for an intimate massage, those on the aphrodisiac list are an obvious first choice. But there are dozens more that are said to have other good effects, relaxing or stimulating or lifting the spirits. (If you really get into this, there are essential oils for practically every human ill.)

It can be a bit baffling when one oil is claimed to be calming, stimulating, antidepressant, energizing and sleep-inducing all at the same time.

Aromatherapists explain that some, like rose and neroli, can stimulate the brain but soothe the nerves at the same time. Others, including geranium and valerian, have a balancing effect, so they'll pick you up if you're feeling down but soothe you if you're tense. Plus different people may experience the effects differently.

How do you know if an all-rounder like ylang ylang or neroli is going to give you added energy or send you off to sleep just when you don't want to? The only answer is to try them out and see. Remember you can use two or three together.

Some essential oils are particularly good for dry skins: these include camomile, clary sage, lavender, neroli, rose, sandalwood and

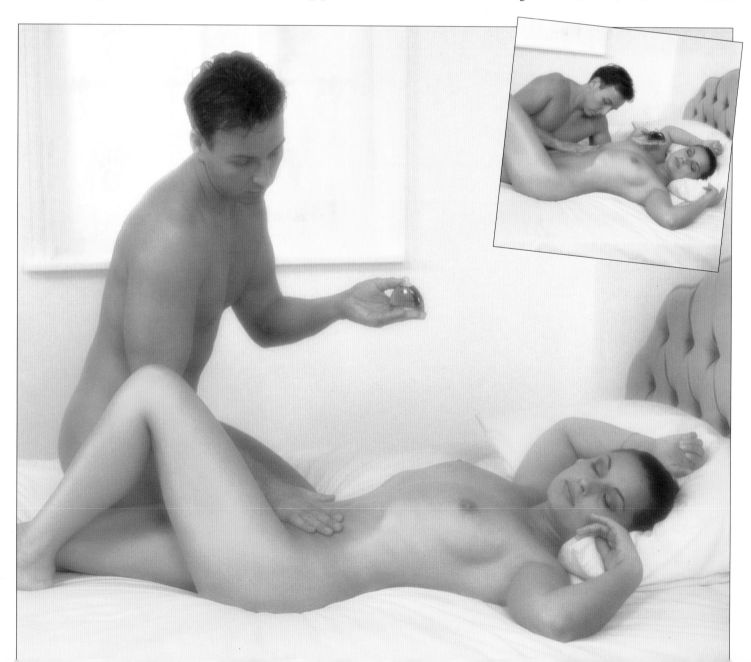

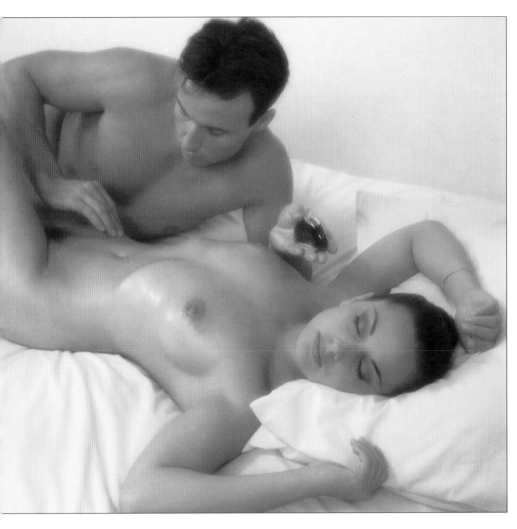

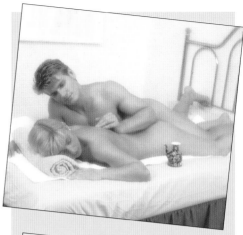

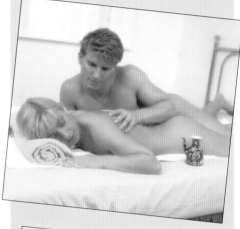

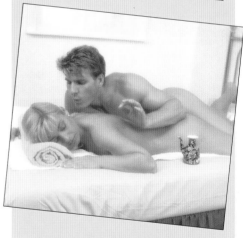

Carefully chosen, the right blend of essential oils could revive you when you're too tired to join in or help you to relax when you're feeling tense or moody.

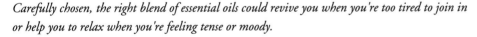

ylang ylang. Frankincense, rose and sandalwood are kind to older skin. For oily skin you could include bergamot, cedarwood, cypress, frankincense, geranium, juniper, lavender, patchouli or rosemary. If your partner suffers from spots, try some camomile, cedarwood, juniper, lavender, patchouli, rosemary or vetivert.

If the night is young but you're feeling jaded, these may give you a burst of energy: benzoin, cardamom, cedarwood, clary sage, coriander, geranium, jasmine, juniper, lavender, marjoram, neroli, patchouli, rose, rosemary, rosewood (bois de rose), valerian or the ever-helpful ylang ylang.

Stressed? Relax with oils of anise, bay, benzoin, bergamot, cajeput, calamus, calendula, camomile, caraway, carrot seed, clary sage, cypress, frankincense, geranium,

hawthorn, heliotrope, jasmine, juniper, lavender, lime, marigold, marjoram, melissa (lemon balm), neroli, opoponax, patchouli, petitgrain, rose, rosewood, sandalwood, taget, valerian, vanilla, vetivert, violet leaf, yarrow or ylang ylang.

If you've had a rough day and you need cheering up, add some of these to your massage: benzoin, bergamot, camomile, clary sage, coriander, frankincense, geranium, jasmine, lavender, marjoram, melissa, neroli, patchouli, petitgrain, rose, sandalwood or ylang ylang.

And when you want to drift quietly off to sleep, use benzoin, bergamot, camomile, clary sage, cypress, frankincense, geranium, jasmine, juniper, lavender, melissa, myrrh, myrtle, neroli, patchouli, rose, sandalwood or, yes, ylang ylang.

The way you use oils has an effect too. If she's in the mood for love but can hardly keep her eyes open, try a mix of sensuous squeezes and featherlight fingertips running up her skin.

For him, smooth some into your breasts, then rub them all over him without letting him move his hands.

These are guaranteed reminders that bed's not just for sleeping in.

Safe & Sensual

If you follow a few simple safety rules, massage will do nothing but good. Essential oils should always be mixed with a carrier oil before touching the skin, as they can have strong effects. For the same reason, don't put them in your mouth. Use twice as much base to dilute the stronger oils – these include cedarwood, camomile, melissa, geranium, neroli, ylang ylang and any citrus oil.

Massage is generally a good thing, but in a few cases including certain cancers, hardened arteries or ulcers, it can be unsuitable. So if you suffer from any health condition check with your doctor that neither massage itself nor aromatherapy oils could do you any harm. (If your doctor's not sure about the oils, just use base oil or the simple ready-blended versions you can buy in beauty shops.) If you have epilepsy or high blood pressure, you should consult a qualified aromatherapist before using essential oils.

All the oils on these lists are normally harmless, but if anything irritates your skin you should wash it off at once. If you use bergamot or any other citrus oil, shower it off before going out in the sun as it could leave your skin more sensitive to burning.

Long nails may look elegant but short ones are much kinder for massage. Always use the pads of your fingers rather than the tips, and keep checking with your partner that you're not hurting. A trained masseuse may press painfully hard on a knotted muscle to break down spasm – but don't try this at home.

Some important safety points are; don't press directly on the spine or joints, and don't massage sore or damaged skin, varicose veins, any inflamed area or a new sprain. Obviously, don't use hacking or drumming moves on the breasts, abdomen or kidneys (on the back below the ribcage). Don't forget to take care of your own muscles when you're doing a massage. Pushing with your hands is exhausting so use the weight of your body instead, and press down through your arms.

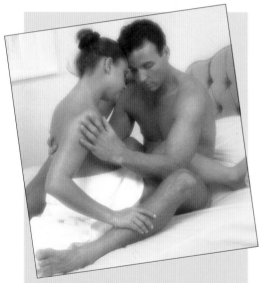

Remind your partner to say at once if anything is uncomfortable, but ask too if you're concerned you may be pressing too hard.

Check occasionally that your partner is warm enough; if not (and it's easy to get cold lying still when the other person is putting some energy into massaging), cover the parts you're not working on with a towel.

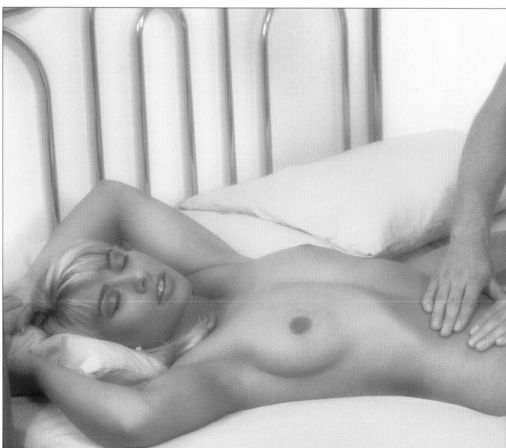

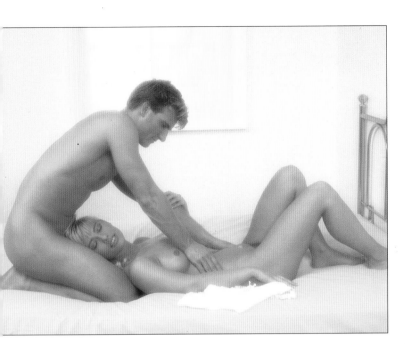

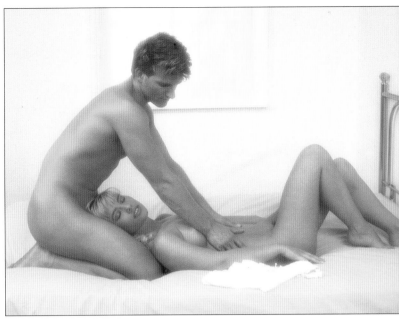

Above left and right: Safety in massage is largely a question of common sense. Don't press anywhere that hurts. Avoid joints and broken skin. Check with a doctor if either of you has a health problem.

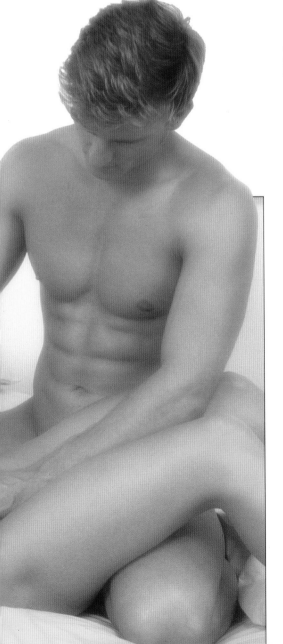

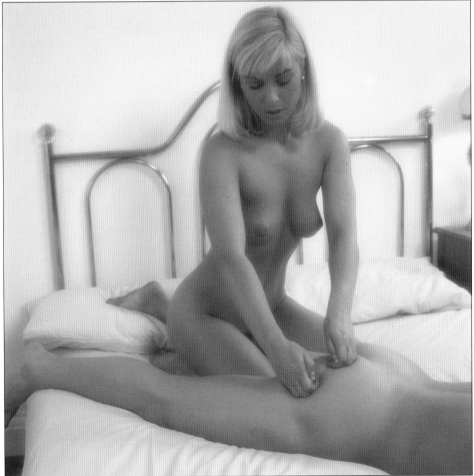

Above: Erotic massage is about light, teasing moves and deeper sensual strokes. Intersperse these with enough pressure to loosen knotted muscles, but without really hurting.

Oil-free Massage

What if you just don't like the feel of oil on your skin? You can still enjoy an all-body erotic massage using fewer techniques.

Although most people enjoy being massaged, some don't like the thought of oil being rubbed into their skin. Luckily, many massage techniques can be done without oil. You only need the lubrication when you're rubbing your hand or fingers across the other person's skin, to prevent an uncomfortable dragging feeling. The same, of course, when you're massaging with other parts or with your whole body!

One compromise is to use body lotion, though this rubs in faster than oil. Some people are happy with talcum powder instead. Otherwise, techniques that don't require lubrication include the thumb-pressure moves such as those used for head massage. (Even if you are using oil, wipe it off before working on the scalp because most people dislike the feel of it in their hair.)

Shiatsu, a type of oriental massage pressing into various points around the body, is done entirely without oil. Another form of traditional Chinese massage includes drumming with the fists on some of the big muscles that hold a lot of tension. And Swedish massage includes those chopping motions you see athletes enduring in films. Shaking, pressing, pulling, kneading and making circles with the thumbs are all done without moving the fingers across the skin, so these feel OK without lubrication too.

You can give a pretty good all-body massage without any oil, using a smaller number of techniques. Squeeze your lover's feet and gently pull the toes, then the feet for a long leg stretch. Knead the big leg muscles, shake the buttocks, walk your fists up beside the spine, knead the shoulders, stretch the back, do a full head massage and work your way down the front using some more from your stock of techniques. Disliking oil is no reason to miss out on the pleasures of massage.

> *Some of the most playful, erotic techniques don't need any oil — running your fingers over your partner's skin in tiny feathery movements that almost tickle but not quite. It feels tantalizing.*
>
> ❧
>
> *Use your fingernails or the ends of your hair, too, for exquisitely light stimulation.*

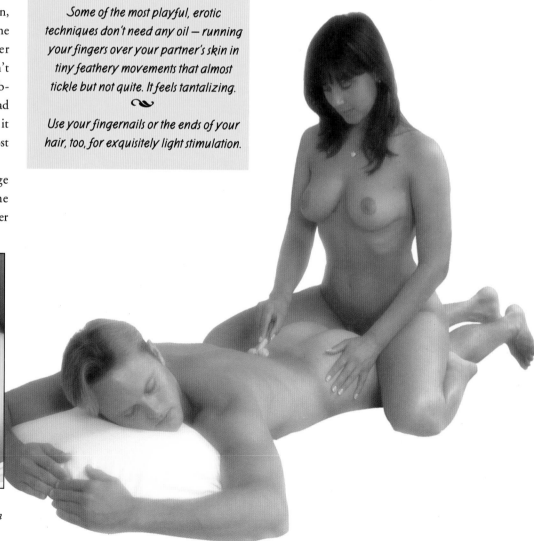

Vary the feel of your massage by using wooden rollers, available with different textures.

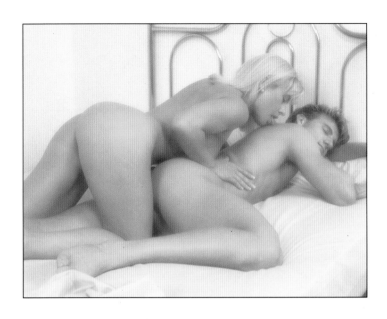

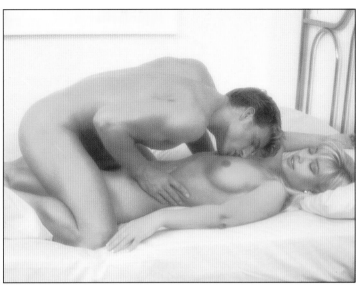

No one wants a mouthful of oil, so make the most of an oil-free massage to try some tantalisingly light moves with your tongue.

Use your tongue to explore your lover's sensitive places – collar bones, nipples, ankles, inner arms, the small of the back.

Try tongue massage both together, lying head to foot with hands clasped behind your back and only the tips of your tongues to explore each other's bodies.

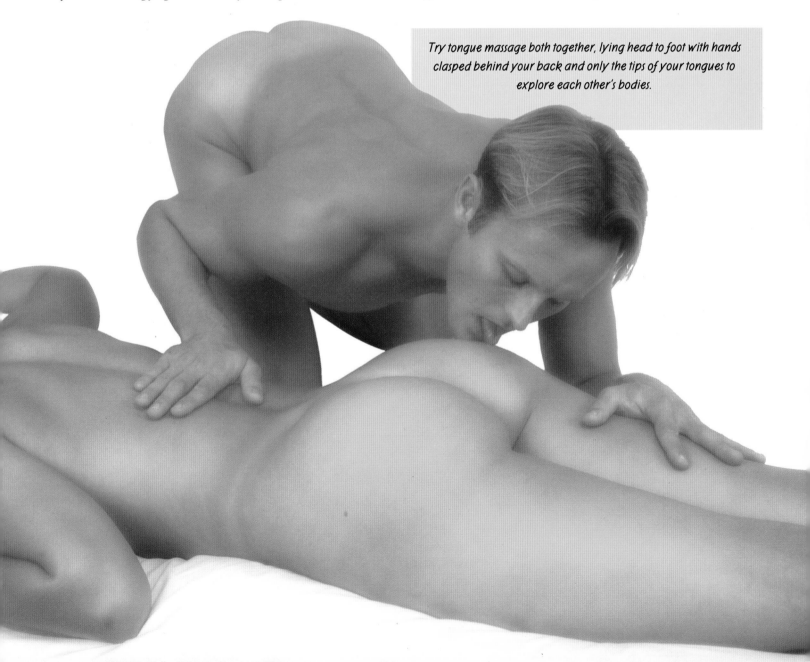

Not Just Hands

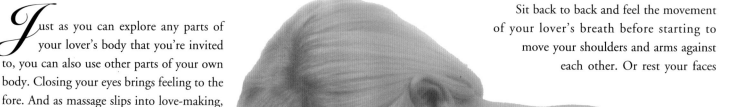

Erotic massage isn't confined by the same limits as other forms of massage. You may find that someone who starts out not liking certain parts of her body touched will soon want to explore all possibilities. You and your lover will be getting to know each other's bodies with an insight and intimacy that's hard to achieve in other ways.

Just as you can explore any parts of your lover's body that you're invited to, you can also use other parts of your own body. Closing your eyes brings feeling to the fore. And as massage slips into love-making, the new moves you'll invent are limited only by your imagination.

A teasing trick any woman can play is to run her nipples lightly over her lover's body. This is a great morale-booster for women who feel their breasts are too small. They'll will be delighted to find size makes no difference at all. The feather-soft touch of fingernails can be equally exciting.

If you have long hair, kneel over your lover and let the ends run across his skin – another teasingly light touch. Short hair can have a more stimulating but equally enjoyable effect for both of you, brushed against the skin and moving over the scalp at the same time. Lips and tongues are among our most sensitive body parts, so running these lightly over your lover's body is another pleasure you can share.

Sit back to back and feel the movement of your lover's breath before starting to move your shoulders and arms against each other. Or rest your faces

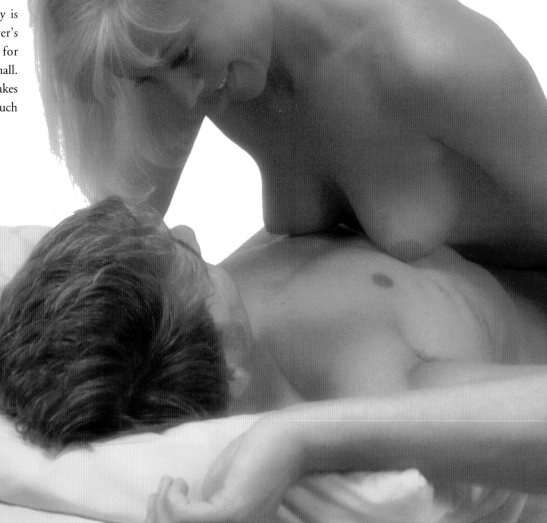

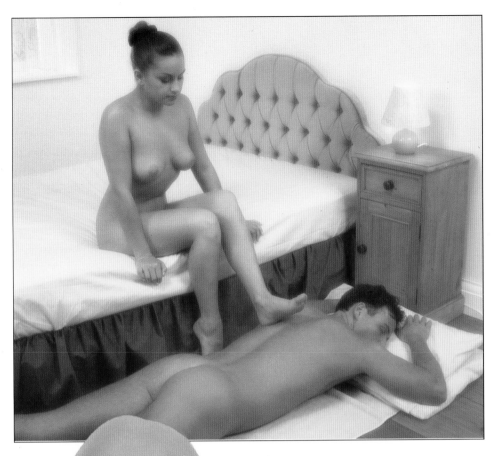

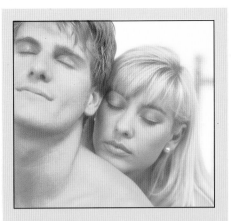

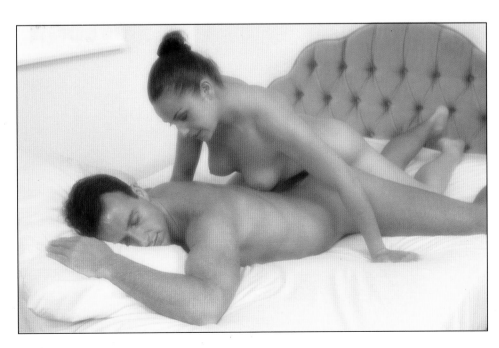

Feet can be as sensitive as hands, backed with the strength of your legs for a deeper massage.

Closing your eyes and touching with other parts of the body gives you a whole new perspective on your lover's body and the sensitivity of your own.

Go all the way and use your whole bodies to massage each other at the same time. As you glide sensuously over your lover's body, feel with your inner thighs, your nipples, the back of your neck. Enjoy the ripple of your partner's muscles, the press of skin to skin and the delicate trail of hair or fingertips.

together with eyes closed and explore the feel of your lover's ears, eyes, cheeks, lips.

For fun, try massaging his back with your feet – heel circles can give a powerful massage and toes can grip surprisingly.

Explore your lover's feet with your own just as you might stroke each other's hands. 'Walk' over each other as you lie side by side. Notice how the soles stop feeling ticklish when you're using them this way.

Bath Games

*A lazy bath is a good way to prepare for a massage.
Lie back and feel the warmth enticing you to forget the stresses
of the day, ready for the pleasures of the night. Why not make
the most of that sensually perfumed water, slippery with
bath oil? An erotic massage can start right here.*

Slip into the water behind your lover and let her relax, leaning against your chest. While your hands are still dry, run your fingers through her hair, first teasing her scalp with your fingertips then pressing with your palms as you move them away from the hairline. Go on to longer moves, stroking her face and neck upwards before reaching her hair. Rub some bath oil into your palms and slowly run them down her sides, cradling her hips, and circling up over her abdomen to her breasts. Feel these floating on the water, lift them gently and continue the smooth stroking movement up to her throat.

Cross your arms to bring your hands down her arms and hold her in a warm hug for a moment before bringing your hands up to the back of her neck. Warm and relaxed by the water, the neck and shoulder muscles will soften readily with your gentle touch.

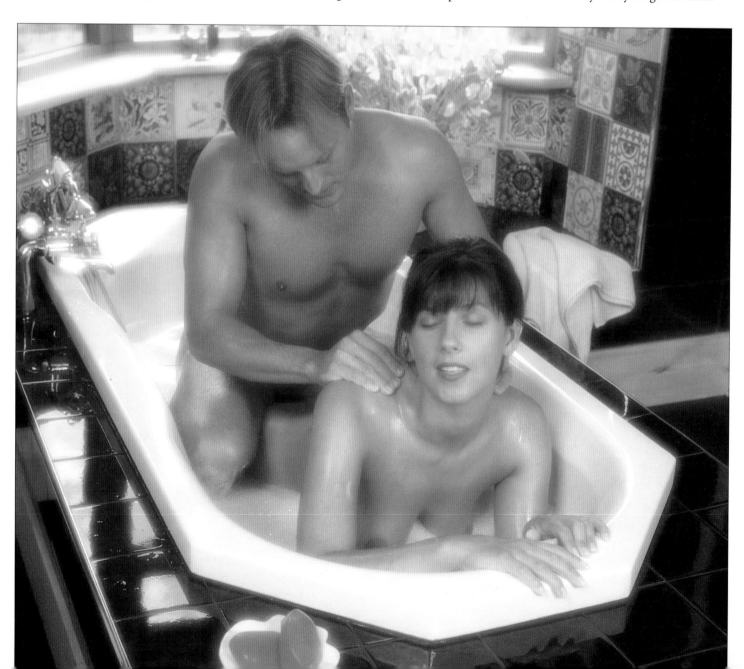

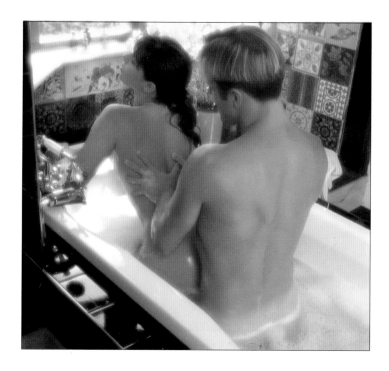

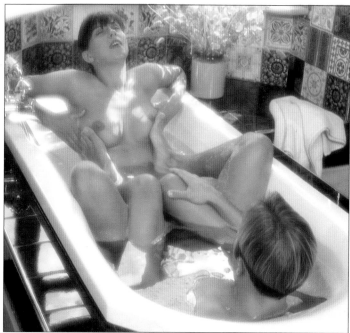

Enjoy the exotic, steamy atmosphere of a headily scented bath.

You don't even need oil – soap is ideal for slippery skin games.

After that, the moves are up to you. Try any of the stroking or kneading moves described in detail on the techniques pages, but aim for long, slow moves that work with the languid flow of the water. Slide your hands down her flanks and along her inner thighs, brushing her pubic hair very lightly as you pass. Run your fingers gently across her breasts, barely touching, then move your hands down her back, lifting her to stroke her hips and buttocks and continue the flowing movement down the back of her legs. By this time she's sure to be joining in.

Baths offer a wealth of textures to play with. Try different skin brushes, sponges and cloths. Experiment with the slipperiness of soap and the frothiness of shower gels. Run brushes lightly up each other's backs while your nipples and bellies slither against each other through a cloud of bubbles.

Out of the bath, smother yourself with froth and slither over him as he lies on a towel, sliding on a film of soap.

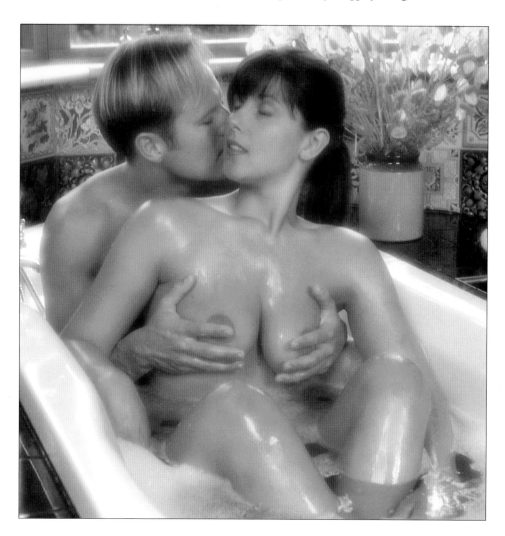

Lapped by the fragrant water, you sink dreamily into your lover's arms.

First Moves

The scene's set, the air is warm and the oil is at room temperature in a bottle or a flattish bowl within reach but not where it's likely to get knocked over. While your lover is undressing you're getting ready too.

Kneel sitting on your heels and straighten your spine as if you're dangling from a string attached to the back of your head. Stretch your arms over your head and bring them down beside you in the biggest circle you can reach. Lift your shoulders up to your ears and let them drop a couple of times till they feel relaxed.

Now practice an important massage movement – lean forward with your chest, keeping your spine straight (instead of leading with the head so you hunch up) and try the same movement to the side and in a circle. Your lower legs need to be anchoring you firmly so you don't lose balance. Positioning your legs securely will help you use your body weight for the movements that need firm pressure to ease tension out of the muscles – a light touch may just feel irritating. If you learn to use your own body weight correctly you'll avoid pressing down from your wrists, which will quickly exhaust you as well as being much less effective. And if you lift up and lean forward in balance from the hips you will ensure you do not end up with a very unromantic backache.

Change your position when you need to, so you're not leaning past your centre of gravity – this can be both uncomfortable and ineffective since you won't be able to control your movements.

Depending on what you're doing you may find it easiest to kneel facing your partner's side, at her head or alongside her, facing her head or feet. You may want to put one knee or foot on the floor to work from a higher position when working on a larger area.

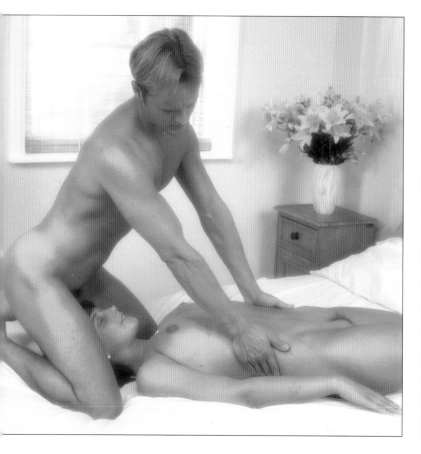

Keep your weight well back on your legs so you're stably anchored and won't lose your balance as you slide your hands forward.

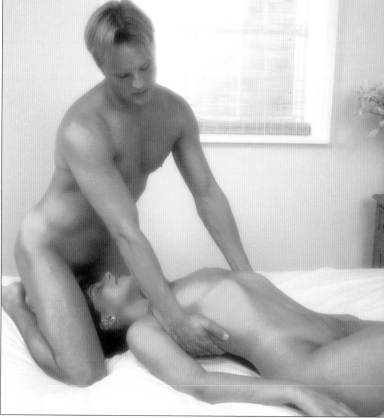

With your back straight and spine lengthened, you can reach farther while still using enough pressure to give an effective massage.

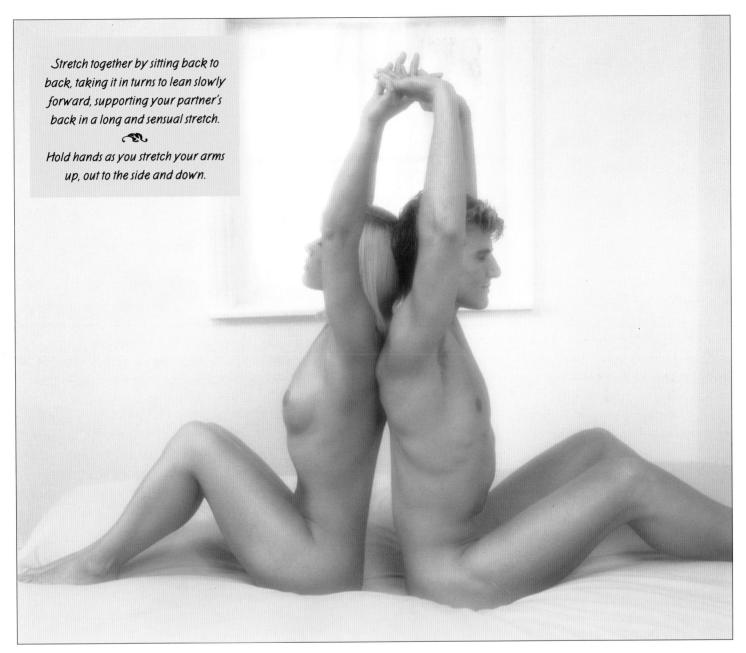

Stretch together by sitting back to back, taking it in turns to lean slowly forward, supporting your partner's back in a long and sensual stretch.

Hold hands as you stretch your arms up, out to the side and down.

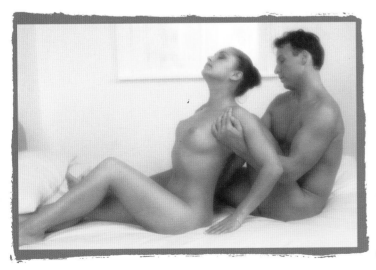

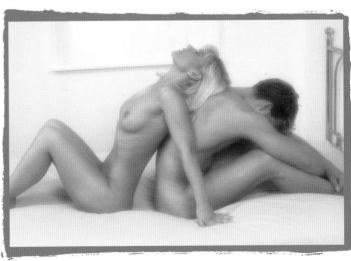

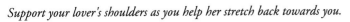

Support your lover's shoulders as you help her stretch back towards you.

This builds the feeling of trust and intimacy between you.

Massage Movements

Any kind of firm rubbing movement helps ease muscle tension and improve circulation. We do it automatically when something hurts. Having a range of techniques adds variety and lets you tailor your style to your partner's needs.

Big muscles take more heavy work than, say, the delicate structures of hands and feet which may need gently flexing and pulling. But don't be put off by techniques that may look complicated or take a bit of practice. The most basic stroking movements are valuable in themselves; in fact

you should start and finish work on any part of the body with these.

Erotic massage is the easiest of all, since so much comes naturally once you start exploring the possibilities of touch. Just running your fingertips over your partner's body is a powerful stimulant – all the other

techniques you can learn simply add to the pleasure and variety.

Try to keep all your movements rhythmic and flowing. You may have to stop to consult the book while you're still learning moves, but you can keep one hand on your partner's back or gently continue stroking while you check what to do.

It's a good idea to keep contact with your partner's body all the time. Traditionally this means keeping one hand on his back while you change position, rearrange towels to keep him warm or reach for the oil. But in practice this can be quite difficult when you're aiming for natural,

Below: A criss-crossing movement on the back helps muscles relax.

> You don't have to learn all the techniques presented here. They're just suggestions – you can try all of them at various times, keep to a few favourites or make up your own.
>
> ❧
>
> A long stroke with both hands can be followed by one with the tongue. Thigh muscles can be kneaded first with your hands, then with your own thigh muscles.

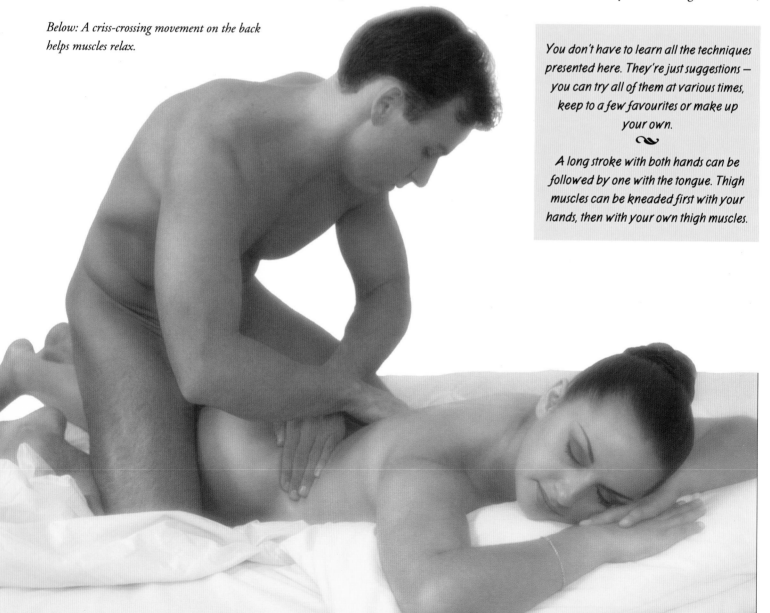

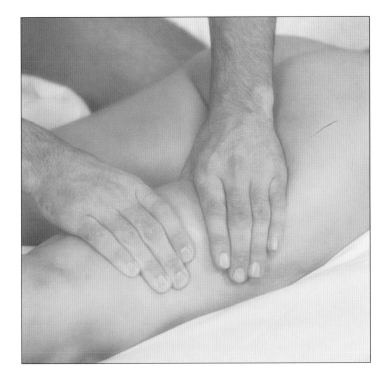

Above: An intimate touch as you start work on your lover's thighs.

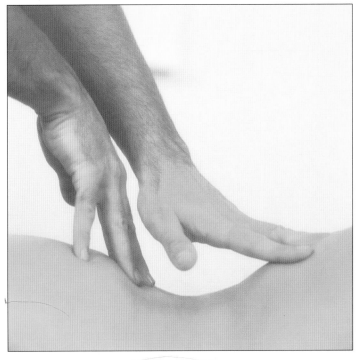

Above: Arouse her with a light reverse stroke down the back.

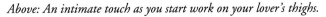

Erotic massage is about having fun, not passing an exam, so it's free to end in wild laughter or wild sex.

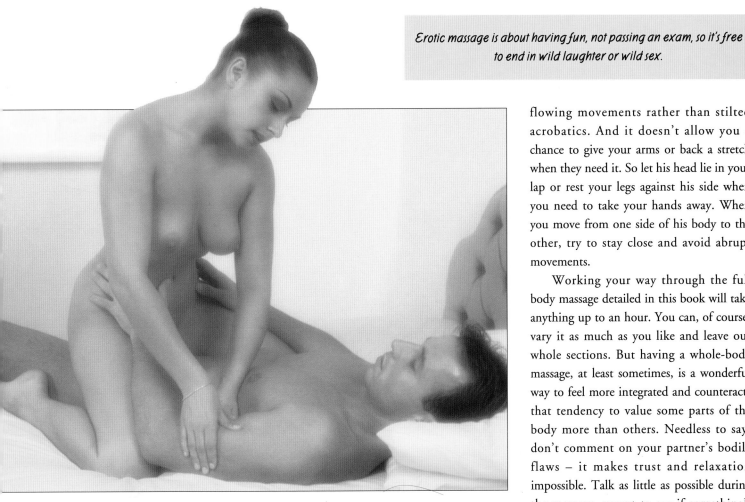

Above: Four hands can work together to share the magic of erotic touch.

flowing movements rather than stilted acrobatics. And it doesn't allow you a chance to give your arms or back a stretch when they need it. So let his head lie in your lap or rest your legs against his side when you need to take your hands away. When you move from one side of his body to the other, try to stay close and avoid abrupt movements.

Working your way through the full body massage detailed in this book will take anything up to an hour. You can, of course, vary it as much as you like and leave out whole sections. But having a whole-body massage, at least sometimes, is a wonderful way to feel more integrated and counteracts that tendency to value some parts of the body more than others. Needless to say, don't comment on your partner's bodily flaws – it makes trust and relaxation impossible. Talk as little as possible during the massage, except to say if something's uncomfortable. Focus on feeling.

Stroking

Stroking is the most basic massage technique, in which the hands slide over the skin and can be used anywhere on the body. Use relaxing stroking moves to start and finish work on any part of the body. For a more stimulating effect, make them faster and lighter.

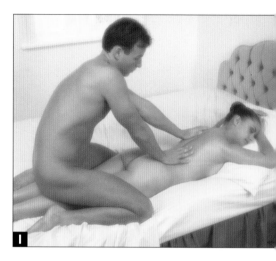

1. Fingers follow where the waist arches, with a teasingly light touch.

Stroking is also known as *effleurage,* since French is the international language of massage. Stroking techniques are firmer on the outward move and light coming back, but you can experiment to find the best pressure.

A very light touch is stimulating rather than relaxing and can be ticklish. Too light a touch may be irritating instead of soothing, so ask your partner how it feels. But the dream touch (page 47) is meant to be tantalizingly light, adding an erotic charge.

Tandem stroking

With hands flat on the skin, fingertips leading, rub firmly away from you. Come back, heel of hand leading, with a gentler stroke. Both hands work together and the firmer first part of the movement should, as far as possible, be towards the heart: up the legs, lower back and abdomen but down the neck, shoulders and upper chest. But don't let this stop you carrying out a beautifully long, slow stroke such as all the way up or down the spine.

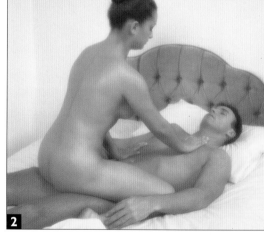

2. Lift each hand when it reaches you, keeping up a flowing movement.

Reverse stroking

Going the opposite direction from tandem stroking: fingers still pointing forward, but you draw your hands gently towards you. Alternate reverse stroking is especially pleasant; bring one hand towards yourself, following with the other when the first hand has nearly reached the end of its journey. Keep doing this in a fluid, circular movement using light pressure. This is a lovely way to complete a massage.

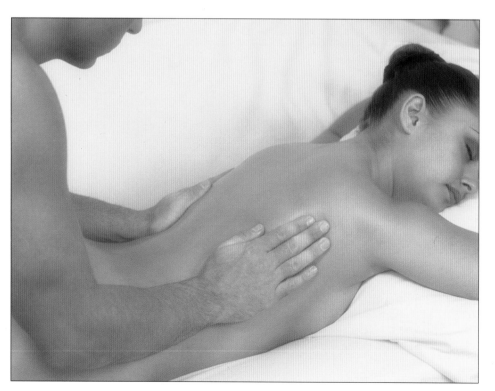

Above: Tandem stroking, with both hands moving up towards your lover's head, is a deep, strong move to start the process of relaxation and arousal.

Cross-stroking

This is a good move on arms and legs. Put one hand above the other across the limb, fingers pointing in opposite directions. Using fairly firm pressure, run the first hand up a short distance and lift it to let the second hand slide up. Continue up the limb with this rhythmic circular movement.

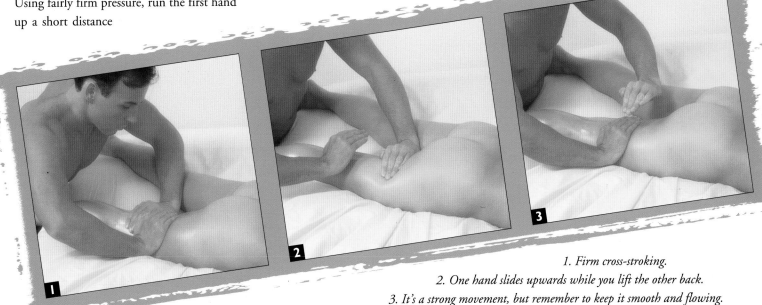

1. Firm cross-stroking.
2. One hand slides upwards while you lift the other back.
3. It's a strong movement, but remember to keep it smooth and flowing.

Circling

This is like the basic tandem stroke, but spreading your hands out to make wide, overlapping circles on a broad area such as the back or abdomen.

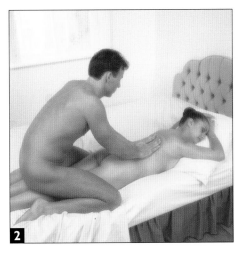

2. Starting right down at the tailbone, run your hands up towards the neck.

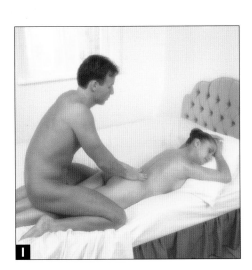

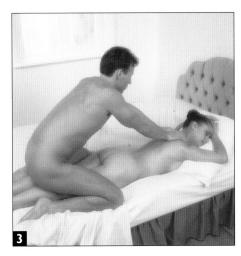

1. Circling is one of the most enjoyable techniques in massage, especially on the back. Deep pressure is relaxing, while a lighter touch could send delicious shivers all the way down her spine.

3. Stroke up over her shoulders before fanning your hands outwards.

4. Bring them back down her sides, pressing gently in and up at the waist.

Deep & Light Stroking

Varying the pressure of a stroking movement gives totally different effects. Deep stroking works on the muscles. Quick light moves are reviving and can be exciting. A feathery touch is intensely stimulating. There's no limit to the number of ways you can enjoy the feel of your lover's body.

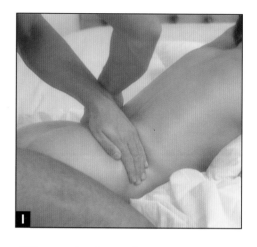

Why not try a change of pace, criss-crossing in a fairly quick rhythm?

Pulling

Put the right hand flat on your partner's skin and pull towards you. As you lift it, start the same movement with the left hand, slightly overlapping the part you have just touched. Use firm enough pressure to move the underlying muscle rather than dragging the skin. Kneeling on one side of your partner's body, work along the opposite side from hip to armpit or up either side of the legs. This has almost the same effects as kneading (page 48), and should follow the initial stroking moves.

Criss-crossing

A variation on pulling. With one hand as before, put your other palm on your partner's near side. Then slide them across the back to change places, passing each other at the spine.

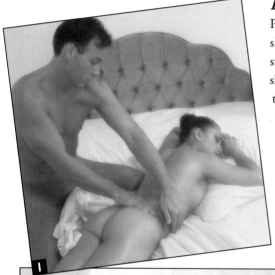

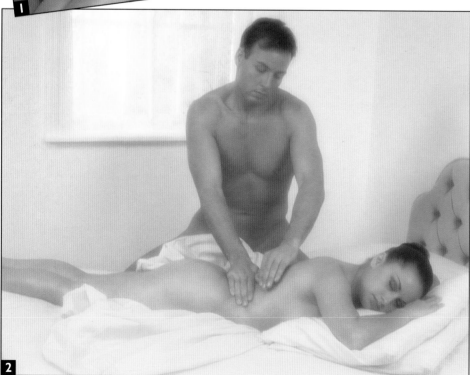

1 and 2 above: Start with fingers tucked underneath for this pulling movement.

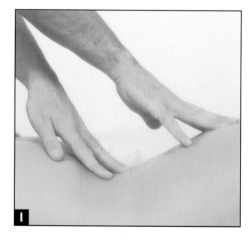

Gentle fingertips alone can exert a light and arousing pressure.

Feathering

Bring the hands towards you with light stroking moves, one at a time but starting each move just before the other has finished. Don't keep stroking one place but work your way out to cover a large area.

Fingernails

A deliciously erotic move. Run your fingers away from you for the lightest touch, or back towards you for a hint of wickedness that's instantly arousing.

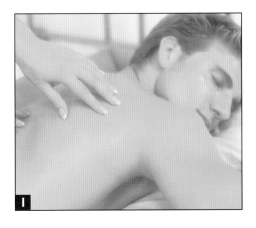

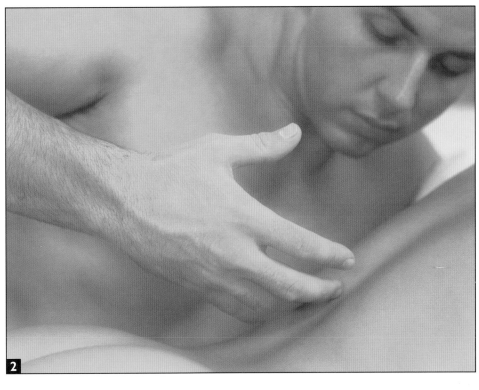

1 and 2: A hint of fingernails adds an edge of shivery excitement.

Dream touch

Run your fingertips lightly, barely touching, the whole length of a limb or around the back or from head to foot. Both hands can work together, mirroring each other's movements or following to create a flowing sensation. This is a stimulating, erotic move. If your partner finds it too ticklish, leave it till later in the massage and try again when he's more relaxed – he's likely to be less sensitive by then. If it's still too light, try a little more pressure.

2. Many of the skills taught in this book can be used outside a seductive setting.

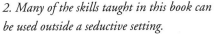

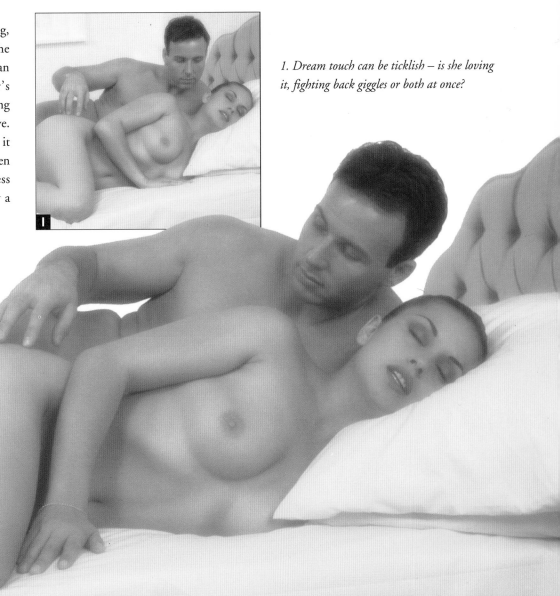

1. Dream touch can be ticklish – is she loving it, fighting back giggles or both at once?

Kneading

Kneading moves have a deeply relaxing after-effect even if they feel a bit strenuous while you're receiving them. If you're aiming for a reviving massage you can make some of them lighter and quicker, more like plucking.

In kneading, or *petrissage*, the hands grip firmly in one place to wring tension out of muscles. These moves can be used on any fleshy or muscular areas, avoiding anywhere bony. Basic kneading and knuckling follow naturally on from the initial stroking moves to start working on the muscles.

Kneading

Pick up as much of the flesh as possible and knead it like bread. Press firmly with the palms side by side; knead rhythmically with the fingers of first one hand then the other. Be careful not to pinch or let the hands slide. This technique works very well on any large area of flesh or muscle, especially the top of the shoulders.

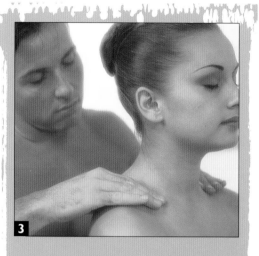

3. Neck and shoulders love to be kneaded.

1. Knead large muscles firmly, using your whole hand.

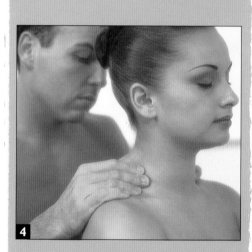

4. Take a big enough grip to hold muscles.

2. Pause to make loving contact before spreading your thumbs out to knead.

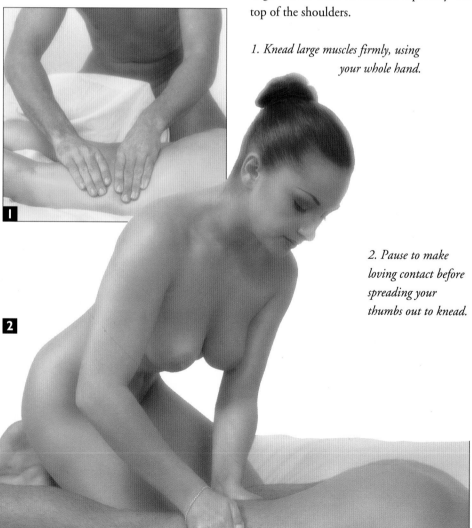

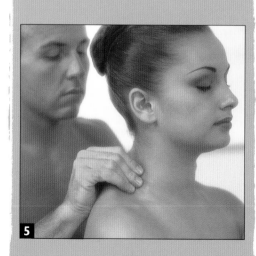

5. Without dragging the skin or pinching, knead tension out of the muscles.

Squeezing

Just as it sounds, squeeze a handful of muscle (or the soft parts of fingers and toes) and quickly let go.

1. A gentle squeezing movement feels good along the upper arms.

2. Lift the skin and muscle.

3. Be careful not to dig your fingers in.

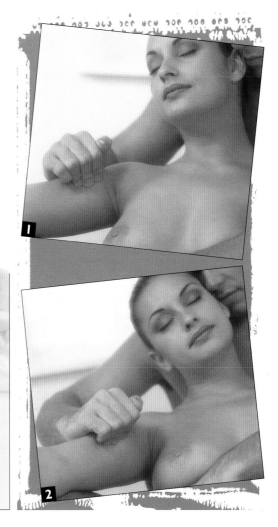

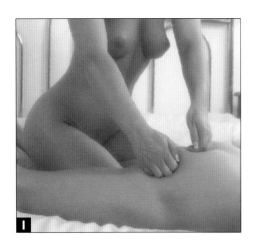

Knuckling

Rest your fists on your partner's skin, knuckles down, and 'knead' with the middle sections of the fingers in circling movements. Check if your partner's enjoying this or feeling mangled.

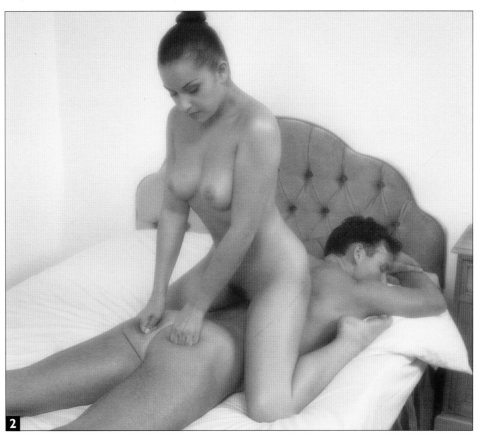

1 and 2. Knuckling is a more strenuous version of kneading, for knotted muscles or if he's dozing off.

Kneading Variations

As you continue to massage your lover you will learn to explore the texture of her skin – admiring her soft curves and resilient muscles, as you slowly uncover the landscape that makes her individual and special.

Plucking

A light, almost teasing variant, this involves lifting small sections of flesh between fingers and thumb and pulling gently before letting go. Use it on fleshy areas such as the thighs, hips and upper arms and on muscular shoulders to release tension. It's a stimulating move, good for waking your partner up if it's all been getting a bit too relaxing.

Picking up feathers

A lighter, faster variation of plucking. Using featherlight pressure with one hand then the other, quickly spread your fingers and thumb then pull them together as if gathering and picking something off your lover's skin. You'll hear a series of brushing sounds interspersed with taps as your thumbs hit your fingers. Another enlivening move.

Wringing

A stronger form of kneading with more of a twist, as if you're wringing out a wet towel. Like all the stronger massage techniques this is excellent for relieving muscle tension. But if you get it wrong it feels like a terror tactic of the school playground.

You could try very gently and see if your partner wants more, maybe to relieve kinked muscles after some heavy work. Use it instead of pulling along your partner's sides, if he's used to massage and wants some deeper work.

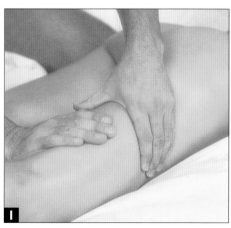

1. Wringing is a powerful move.

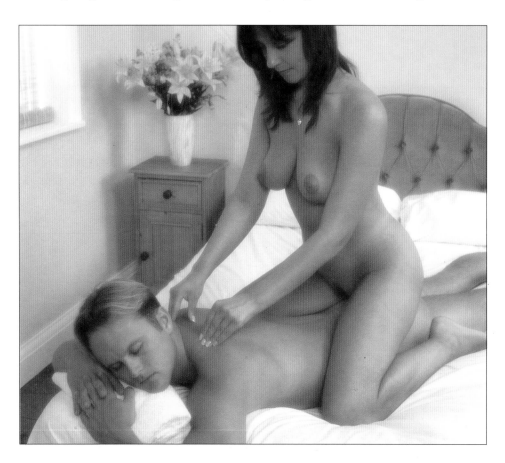

Above: Plucking and picking up feathers are sexy, stimulating techniques. They're among the few moves that feel good anywhere, even over bony areas.

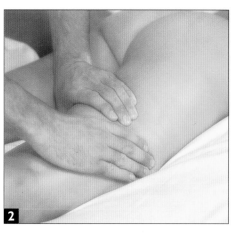

2. It can revive tired muscles after a workout, but take it gently at first.

Skin-rolling

Taking a handful of flesh in each hand, walk the fingers back towards the thumbs but stop before the movement becomes a pinch. Work your way over large fleshy or muscular areas this way.

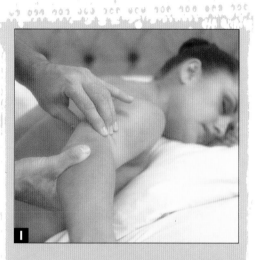

1. In skin-rolling, each finger counts.

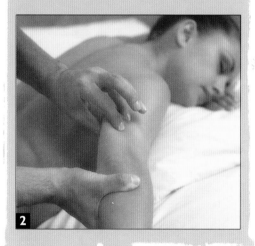

2. Imagine playing a perfect instrument.

Right: Shake out tension, with firm pressure over a muscle or gently when holding a hand or a foot.

Gripping

Hold a handful of flesh with fingers on side of the bone, thumb the other, and pull them towards each other, for example on the back of the neck, the arms or the front of the thighs. Don't let them slide over the skin, and stop short of pinching.

Right: Gripping is a good move for loosening up. It feels as if you're pulling skin away from bone.

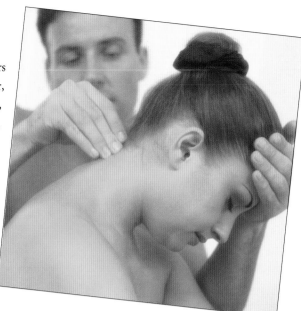

Shaking

This moves the muscles too, though without any kneading pressure. You can shake arms and legs very gently, to release tension without hurting the joints.

Holding a hand or foot off the floor, gently pull and shake the limb before putting it back down. Or spreading your hand over a large muscle – say the buttocks or legs – give it a vigorous shake for a few seconds. This is a playful, stimulating movement that can arouse your partner ready for action.

Friction

Like the kneading techniques, these work to wring tension out of muscles. But friction involves movement across the skin, so you need enough oil to avoid dragging the skin without making it too slippery. These work more deeply on the muscles, so they can be used instead of kneading.

As with all massage movements, be sure to do this with relaxed shoulders, trying to use body weight instead of tensing up your wrists and hands. Massage is meant to release tension, not just transfer it from one person to the other!

Many people often start by liking only the gentlest massage techniques, but as they get used to the feel, they come to enjoy the relaxing after-effects of a deeper massage.

Since you're doing this for pleasure, stick to the techniques you both like for a relaxing experience, and try out others when you're both feeling adventurous. You may be surprised at how wonderful the deeper massage movements can feel.

Thumb-rolling

Press hard with the pads of the thumbs (not the tips) and run them up a muscle, either both together in a long stroke or one after the other in an overlapping motion. This is ideal for the long muscles of the back and legs, which often hold so much tension they need a whole variety of methods to get them really relaxed.

Hand friction

Pressing with the heel of one hand, rub a short distance up the muscle. Lift that hand as the other hand starts the same move, going slightly further up.

This is useful on large, long muscles such as in the calves and thighs.

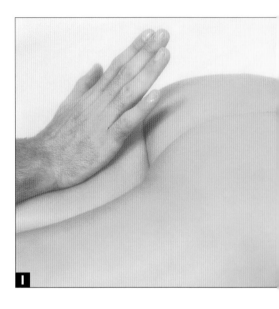

1. Hand friction – or is this just doing what comes naturally?

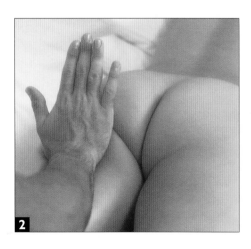

2. Rub firmly upwards with one hand or both alternately, using plenty of oil so your hand slides instead of catching.

1. Thumb-rolling releases tightness from long muscles. Press firmly with the fleshy pads of your thumbs, enjoying the long smooth glide.

2. Keep up a fluid rhythm, one thumb starting its work as you lift the other and bring it down in a circular movement.

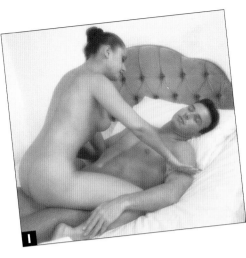

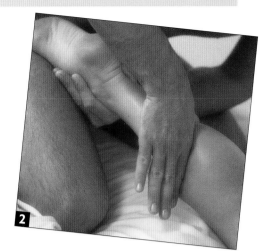

Rubbing

This is like stroking but with more pressure, often using the web between thumb and first finger.

2. Rubbing like this can wring the knots out of a very tight muscle …

3. … but it can feel odd. Sexy or strange? Try it and see what you think.

1. The web between finger and thumb exerts a surprising amount of pressure.

4. If you both enjoy the feeling, use it to slide up your lover's arms or legs.

4

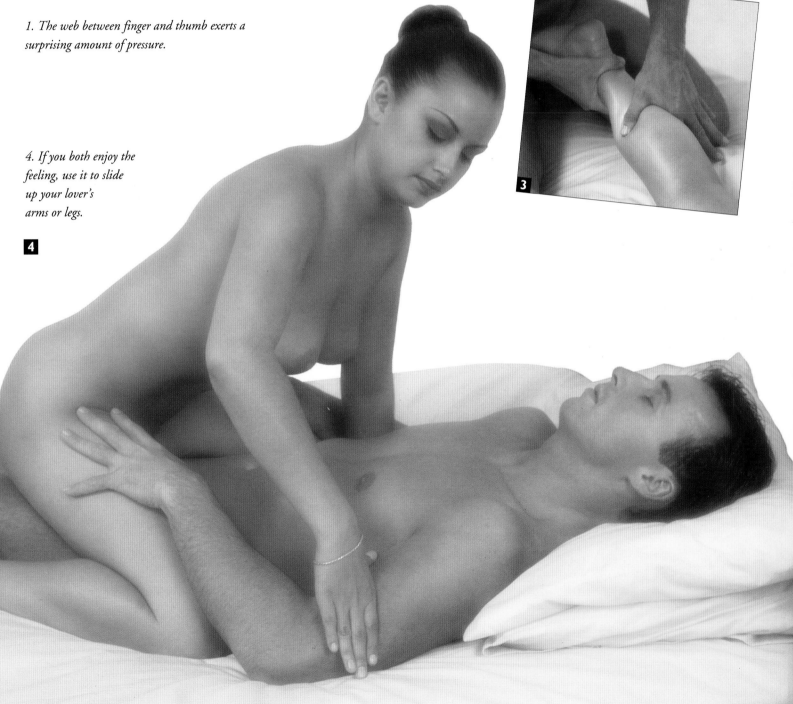

Pressure

In an erotic massage, pressure is used now and then to vary the stroking and kneading moves. It's also useful if one of you feels too tired and achy to enjoy sex, since it's a good way of breaking down muscle tension. Press hard on one spot, either straight down or making small circling movements.

Fist pressure

Make loose fists and put the backs of your fingers (from knuckles to lowest joint) on a tight muscle. Lean with straight arms for more pressure. This is a static movement – the moving version called knuckling doesn't press so deeply.

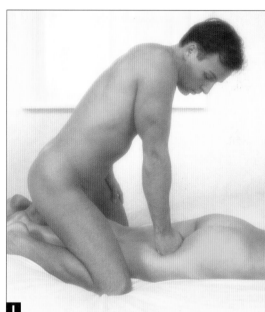

1. Strong pressure can help ease tension out of overworked muscles.

*I*t's safe to try reasonable pressure on big, tight muscles but don't persist if it doesn't help. Only do this if your partner asks, since it can be uncomfortable and could leave him feeling more tense than before.

Below: Thumb circles work deeply on large areas of muscle. Find your lover's hidden tensions and help them ebb away.

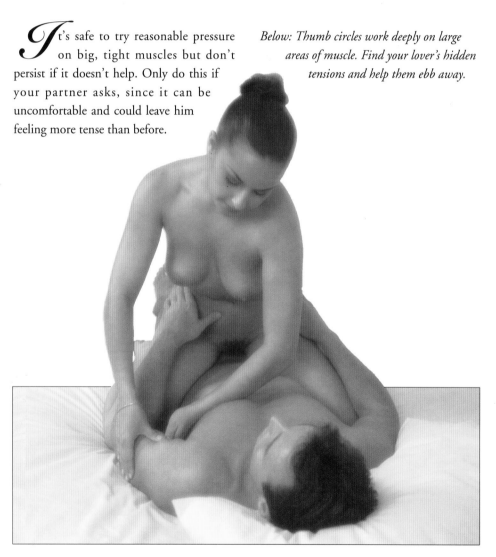

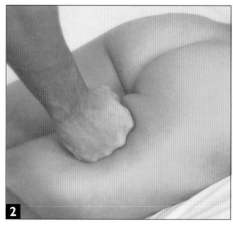

2. Is she enjoying this or enduring it? Remind her to say if anything hurts.

Thumb circles

Pressing firmly with the pads of the thumbs, make little circles in one spot, moving the skin and the muscle below rather than letting the thumbs slide over the skin.

Unlike the shiatsu thumb-pressure described on page 90, these thumb circles use the whole length of the soft pad above the top knuckle of the thumb.

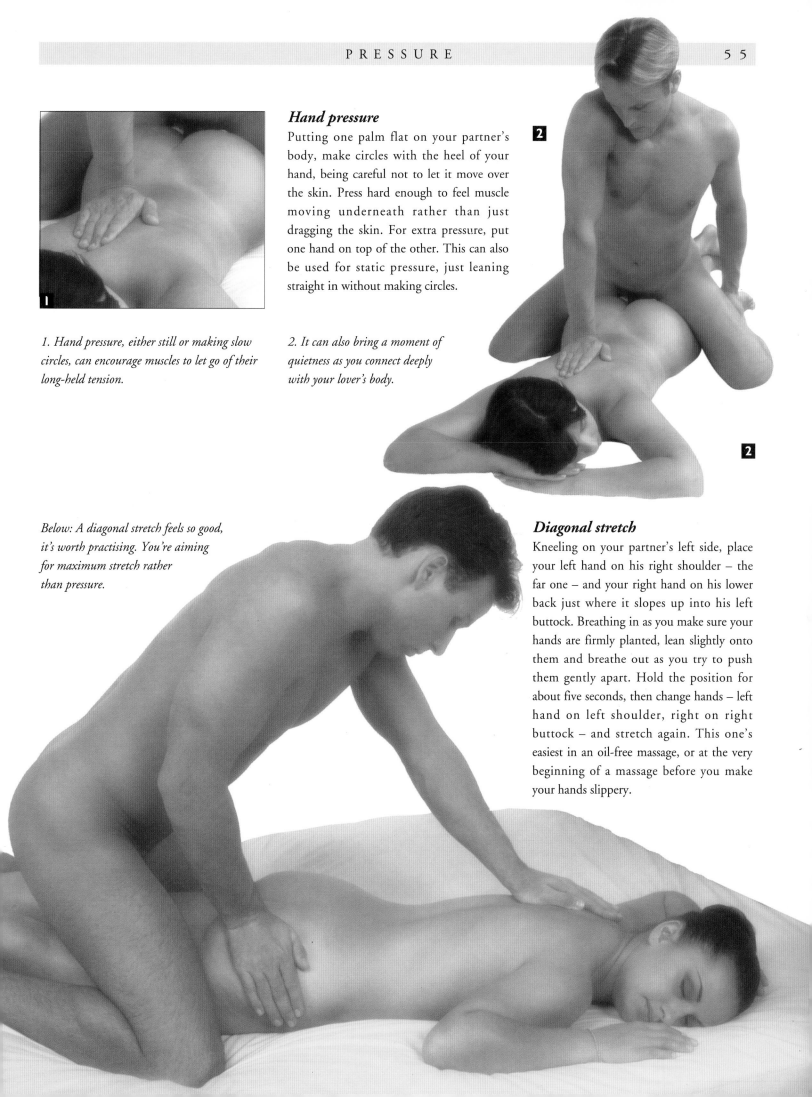

Hand pressure

Putting one palm flat on your partner's body, make circles with the heel of your hand, being careful not to let it move over the skin. Press hard enough to feel muscle moving underneath rather than just dragging the skin. For extra pressure, put one hand on top of the other. This can also be used for static pressure, just leaning straight in without making circles.

1. Hand pressure, either still or making slow circles, can encourage muscles to let go of their long-held tension.

2. It can also bring a moment of quietness as you connect deeply with your lover's body.

Below: A diagonal stretch feels so good, it's worth practising. You're aiming for maximum stretch rather than pressure.

Diagonal stretch

Kneeling on your partner's left side, place your left hand on his right shoulder – the far one – and your right hand on his lower back just where it slopes up into his left buttock. Breathing in as you make sure your hands are firmly planted, lean slightly onto them and breathe out as you try to push them gently apart. Hold the position for about five seconds, then change hands – left hand on left shoulder, right on right buttock – and stretch again. This one's easiest in an oil-free massage, or at the very beginning of a massage before you make your hands slippery.

Percussion

A lively and stimulating technique, percussion means hitting the skin – with light, bouncy movements, not hurting it. Gentle drumming or cupping can be quite relaxing, but faster percussion moves are arousing when sprinkled through an erotic massage.

Although it may look rough, percussion massage (*tapotement*) is excellent for improving the circulation and is actually much milder than the kneading techniques. It's best on the big muscles of the back, legs and buttocks, avoiding bones and joints. Gentle drumming or cupping can be quite relaxing. But faster percussion moves are stimulating – good if your partner looks like drifting off to sleep too soon, or sprinkled through an erotic massage.

Drumming

Make loose fists and gently hit with the ends farthest from your thumbs. This is particularly good for the back as long as you keep away from the spine and the kidneys, just below the ribcage.

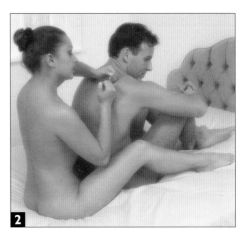

1. Wake him up with some light, loose drumming on his back.

2. A gift from the exotic east: drumming is a Chinese massage technique.

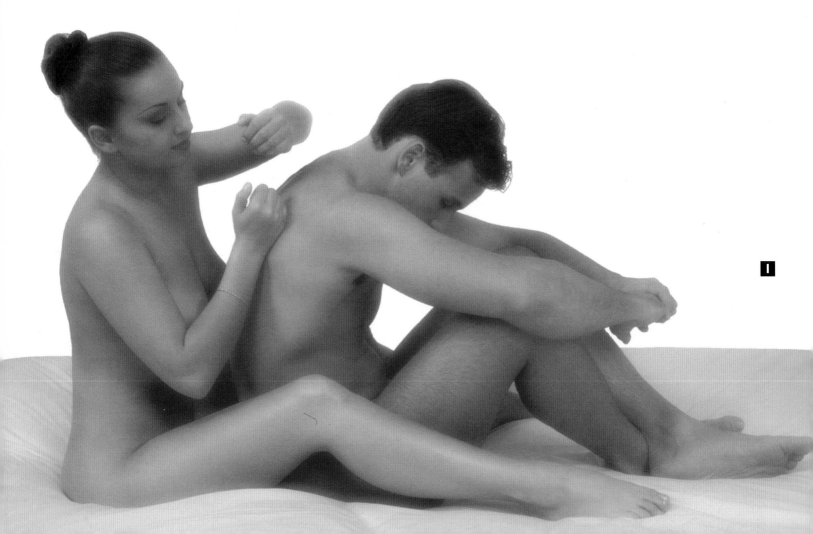

Cupping

Keeping your wrists relaxed, turn your hands down with palms slightly rounded. Bring them down on your partner's skin one after the other at about heartbeat speed – slower than hacking. The sound is slightly muffled since it's mainly air hitting the skin: if your hands were covered in paint they'd leave rings rather than hand-shaped patches.

1. Keep to a steady rhythm, like the sound of a horse's hooves.

2. It looks rough, but it's mainly air that's hitting his skin.

Tapping

Tap with your fingertips, varying the speed and pressure.

Hacking

A series of quick karate-like chops – only much lighter! – on the big muscles, especially of the legs and back. Famous from Swedish massage as seen in films. This one can feel quite sharp as it touches the skin but shouldn't be hard enough to hurt after you've stopped doing it. Be especially careful not to work over the abdomen, kidneys, bones or joints, or even close to them where you'd be hitting ligaments rather than muscle.

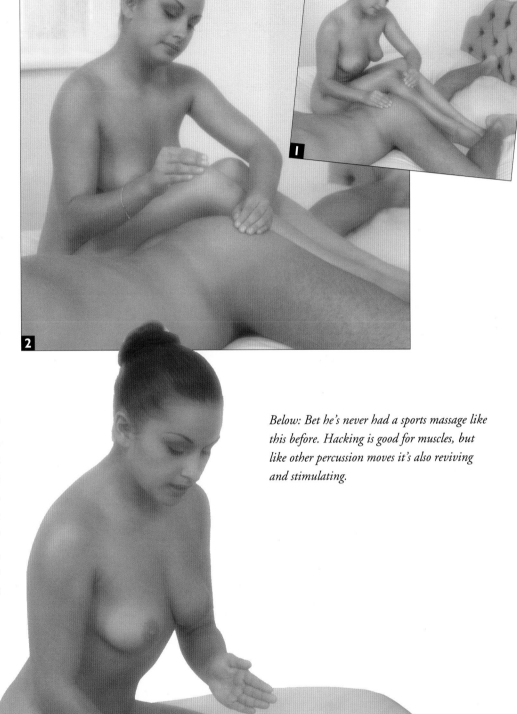

Below: Bet he's never had a sports massage like this before. Hacking is good for muscles, but like other percussion moves it's also reviving and stimulating.

The Back

Make sure your partner is lying comfortably on his front, arms by his side if that feels all right or otherwise pillowing his face. The ideal position for a back massage is lying face down with a small rolled towel supporting the forehead and arms resting by the sides, because this keeps the spine straight.

Kneel by his left side, facing his head. Rub your hands together to warm them, and put them palms-down on his back while you start feeling attuned to his body. Next comes the best moment to do a *diagonal back stretch*, before your hands become slippery with oil: hands on opposite shoulder and buttock, try to push them gently away from each other.

Then pour a small amount of oil into one palm and smooth it into both hands, making sure it's at skin temperature. Close your eyes as you spread it slowly over his back, letting all your awareness move into your hands. Run them over him, feeling the curve of muscles, the sharp plane of bones, the varying texture of skin. Don't press on scars and blemishes, but observe them without criticism. You're starting to know your lover's body in a way you never have before, even in your most intimate moments.

After a while, put your hands palm-down one on each side of his spine, fingers pointing towards his shoulders and start *tandem stroking*. Rub quite firmly from the base of his spine up to the neck in one long, slow move with both hands. Lean forward from the waist as you go so your hands don't get too far out in front or they're likely to slip away suddenly. (If they did, and left you sprawling, or if you had to strain your lower back to stop that happening, you'll see why the right posture is important.)

Trying to keep a flowing movement, bring your hands across the top of his shoulders and back down his sides, pressing in gently as they come back up at his waist. Then repeat the movement, spreading your hands out more to work on his whole back.

Starting from the base of the spine again, rub up beside the spine using your weight to apply more pressure. Hook your hands over his shoulders and pull gently towards you. Bring your hands back down the sides.

Below: Start with the diagonal stretch.
See how her back widens as it loosens up.

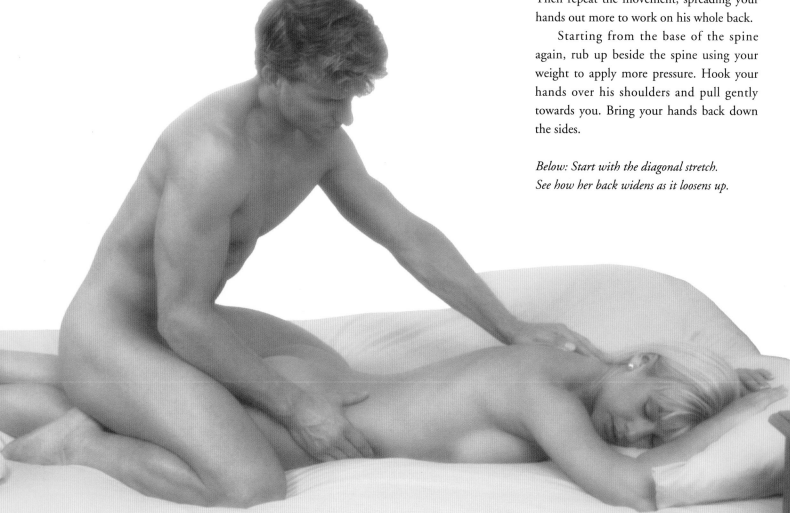

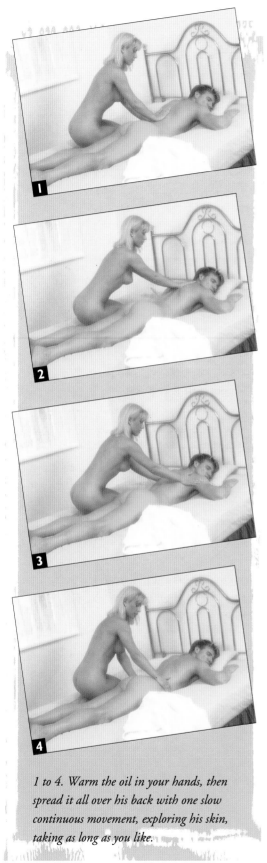

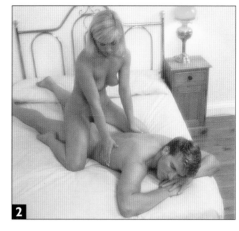

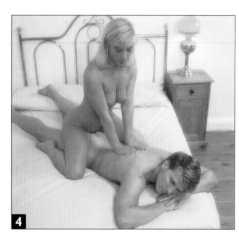

1. Stroke firmly up beside his spine.

2. Bring your hands back down his sides.

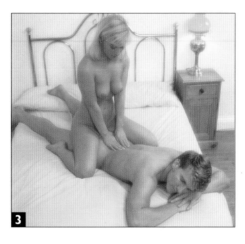

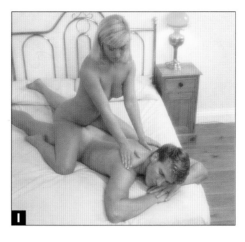

3. Feel the ripple of muscles in his back.

4. Repeat this sequence several times.

1 to 4. Warm the oil in your hands, then spread it all over his back with one slow continuous movement, exploring his skin, taking as long as you like.

Right: Sitting astride him, explore his skin with your thighs as well as your hands.

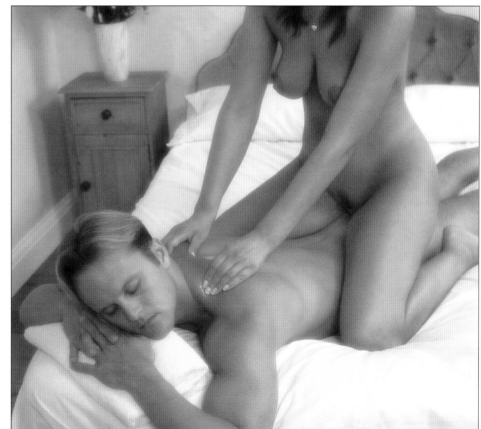

More on the Back

Add oil as soon as you feel skin starting to drag, pouring it into your hands and smoothing it in. Then make sure it's at skin temperature before you touch your partner again.

After several stroking movements up the back, add some *friction*. You will find that **thumb-rolling** is particularly good for releasing tension from the muscles beside the spine. This time, the tips of your thumbs rest beside the spine with your hands slightly further out. The fingers still point towards your partner's head, but the thumbs point inward and just slightly upward. Press into the muscles beside the spine with the sides of your thumbs, running them up to the neck in a long smooth movement. Be sure to press on the long muscles beside the spine, not on the vertebrae themselves.

Light drumming changes the pace of a massage – try it if your soothing movements are sending him to sleep.

When you reach the neck, spread your hands out across the shoulders and bring them back to the base of the spine in the usual way, with a long firm stroke. Repeat this once or twice.

Next, do the same technique slightly differently. Press with your right thumb first, keeping the pressure constant as you slide it up a few inches. Follow on the other side with the left thumb, going slightly further up.

*Making loose fists, gently **drum** all over the back, avoiding the spine. Keep your wrists relaxed so the movement is light and bouncy.*

This is a lively, stimulating move that will wake your partner from a state of dreamy relaxation, ready for anything.

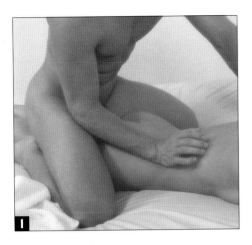

1. *Pressing here with the heel of your hand can ease period pains like magic.*

Repeat the movements in a flowing pattern all the way up to the neck, pressing and sliding with one and then the other. Bring your hands back with a smooth stroking movement to the base of the spine.

Walk your fists gently up beside the spine from the small of the back using *fist pressure*, leaning with straight arms on the backs of your fingers. Remind your partner to say at once if anything hurts, as it's easy to put too much weight into this.

Finish by stroking with both hands up the spine – this feels soothing after the deep pressure.

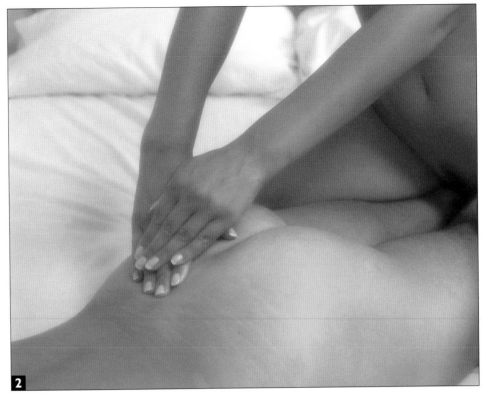

2. *Too light a touch can feel irritating, like being tickled. If you're the smaller partner, you can add pressure by leaning with both hands.*

Try some hand pressure on the lower back, – often the most tired part of the body.

Put one hand over the other and press with the heel of the hand, either straight down or in little circles without moving across the skin. Lift the hands and do the same a couple of inches away, working across the back without leaning on the spine.

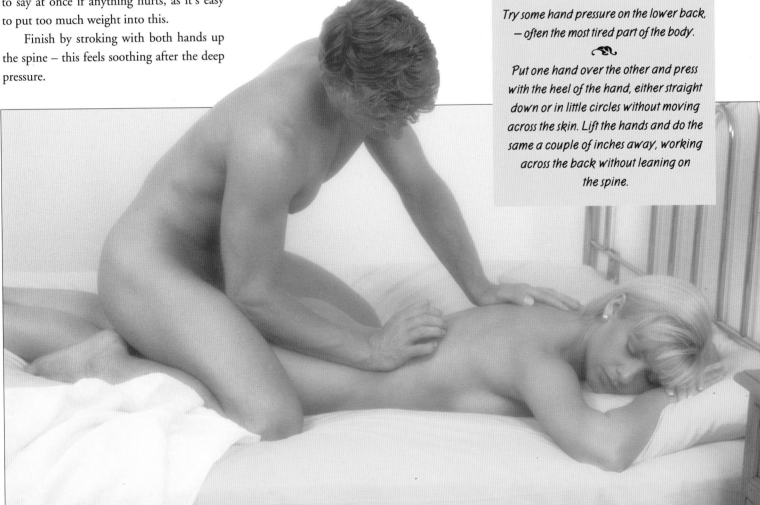

Shoulder Blades & Sides

Kneel alongside your partner and give her a stimulating shoulder blade massage to smooth away the tension of the day. To establish a feeling of greater contact between you, kneel lightly astride her, with your thighs gently brushing her sides.

Find the edge of the left shoulder blade and massage along just under it with little *thumb circles*. For this section, your partner may find she benefits most by lying with arms by her sides. To see the contour of the shoulder blade clearly, gently lift her hand and move the arm, supporting it with your other hand. Lay her hand carefully on the small of her back so the shoulder blade stands out unmistakably; if this is uncomfortable just put the arm back by her side after noting the area you'll be working on.

Massage the area below the edge of the shoulder blade, not on the bone itself. Starting by the outside edge, press the pads of your thumbs under the outer edge of the shoulder blade and make little circles without dragging them over the skin. Lift the thumbs, put them down about a thumb's width along and do the same again, working your way round to the far end of this L-shaped bone. When you have finished, carefully lift your partner's arm off her back and replace it gently beside her or under her head.

Pulling is a gentle way of working on the sides. Kneeling facing her side, reach across and put your right hand flat on her far hip, so your fingertips are near the bed. Pull firmly towards you. As you raise your hand, start the same movement with the left hand an inch or two along towards her waist, slightly overlapping the part you have just touched. Press firmly enough to move the underlying muscle rather than dragging the skin. Work your way up to her armpit, your arms moving in a rhythmic dance.

Moving your hands back to waist level, repeat this pulling movement but make it longer. Bring your hands towards you, with a lighter pressure across the back.

Don't forget to pay attention to the sides when you are massaging your lover's back.

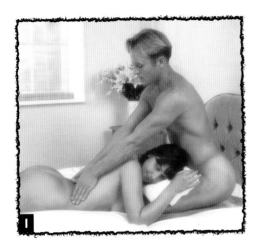

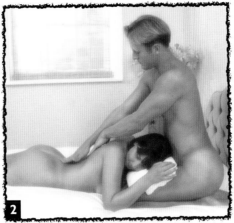

1. Add some variety to a back massage.

2. Try kneeling at your lover's head.

3. Explore the different feelings together.

When this has all become easy, try a **criss-crossing** version that may take a couple of attempts to co-ordinate. With one hand as before (palm flat on her far side, finger-tips near the bed) put your other palm on your partner's near side. Then slide them across her back to change places, an inch or two nearer her waist. They should pass each other at about the spine. Work your way up the back, pressing firmly on the sides and lightly across the spine. When you've finished working on one side, move over and do the same for the other.

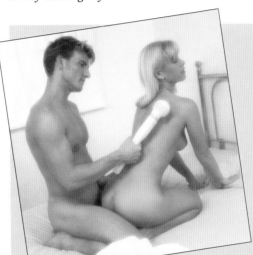

Lighter than the most delicate touch, **blowing** on your lover's skin can make her shiver deliciously. Try blowing down her side or into her hair, following this with a firm stroking movement.

∾

Running your tongue across her skin can have the same erotic effect. Or add some props: an electric massager, a feather duster, the trailing end of a scarf or a vibrator.

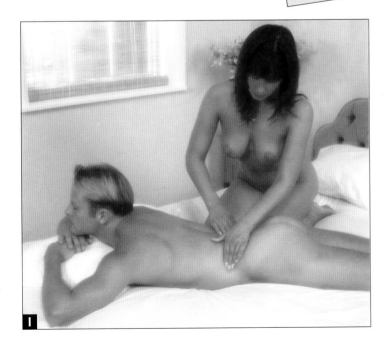

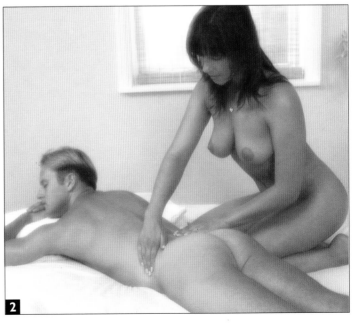

1. Both men and women love having the stress gradually massaged out of their backs.

2. Take time to explore the changing contours of his body as he slowly relaxes under your loving touch.

Completing the Back Massage

Some men love their partners to sit on their buttocks during the back massage. It's actually easier to do some of the movements from there, especially those going up beside the spine. It's fun to try this, and feels very sexy and intimate.

Variations include squatting astride your partner without putting your weight down, which is a wobbly position to give a real massage from but can be a fun way to finish a massage when you have more body contact in mind. You can also try kneeling between your partner's legs, if they're very flexible. Or try it when you're both in more of an 'erotic' mood than a 'massage' mood – you might even find it works for both. Most people enjoy plenty of back massage. Anything up to about half an hour can be good for this area, which bears the brunt of so much stress and tiredness.

You may notice your partner's skin reddening as you work on it with some of the deeper methods such as friction with your thumbs. Don't worry as long as he's comfortable. You're aiding his circulation by bringing blood to the area.

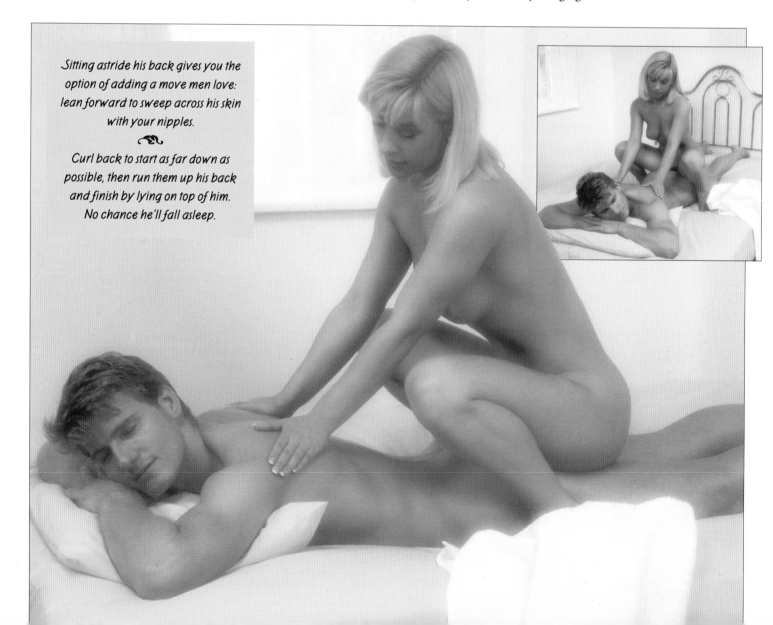

Sitting astride his back gives you the option of adding a move men love: lean forward to sweep across his skin with your nipples.

❧

Curl back to start as far down as possible, then run them up his back and finish by lying on top of him. No chance he'll fall asleep.

If you're both new to massage it's best to start with the gentler movements. Surprisingly, even strong men can wince at having their muscles kneaded if they've never felt this before. If it feels more than slightly sore the next day, you may have gone on too long, especially if your partner isn't used to massage. You won't have done any harm as long as you've followed the safety rules – not pressing directly on the spine or doing anything painful, especially over bones. It's part of the process of discovering each other's bodies, so don't be put off trying again later.

Remember to finish the back massage with some soothing *strokes*. Several long smooth strokes straight up your lover's back will feel good, one hand going up as the other returns, and finishing with some sweeping movements to include the whole back.

*Tease your lover by running your **fingernails** down his sides, just hard enough to excite rather than tickling.*

You can continue this tantalising move over his whole back and up into his hair. It's one of many playful moves you can add to enliven a massage at any point you like.

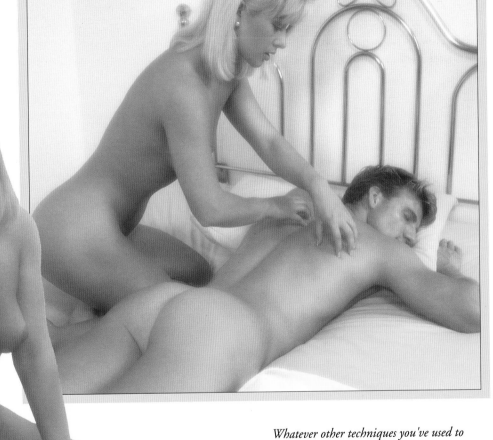

Whatever other techniques you've used to massage your lover's back, finish with some leisurely upward strokes.

Calves

Hold one foot between both hands for a moment, warming it, then lift and gently pull the leg towards you, positioning it comfortably before you start a sensuous calf massage.

our a little oil onto your hands – more if your partner's legs are hairy – and begin massaging the calves. The large muscles of the leg benefit from deep massaging, but be careful not to put any pressure on the knees.

If you start by kneeling at your lover's feet, you can continue however you like. This is a good area for *cross-stroking*. Put your left hand on the calf with fingers pointing right, and the right hand with fingers pointing left, one hand just above the other. Using fairly firm pressure, *stroke* with both hands up the back of his left leg from ankle to buttock in one smooth movement, gliding lightly over the knee. Fan your hands out to glide down the sides of the leg. Repeat the movement with more pressure. Use enough oil to slide smoothly over the hairiest part.

Stroke lightly down to the ankle and *knead* your way up the left calf muscle to just below the knee, grasping and releasing the muscle rhythmically with alternate hands. This is the most comfortable method to use on legs with a lot of hair, since it doesn't involve any pulling. You may find this easier if you shift your position slightly to one side and grasp across the muscle.

Stroking lightly down to the ankle and kneeling at your partner's feet again, work your way up to just below the knee using the *thumb-rolling* technique. Or move up the calf with a series of little *squeezes*, or *rub*

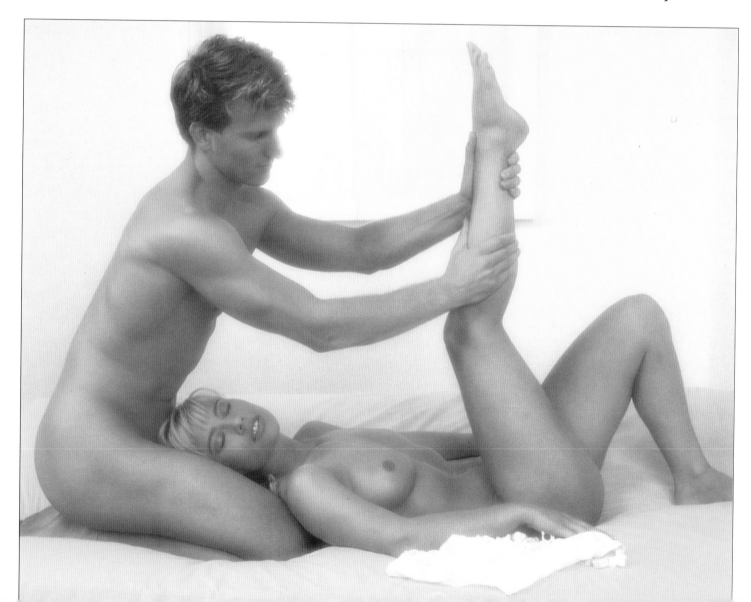

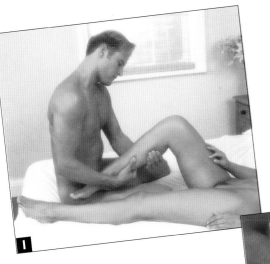

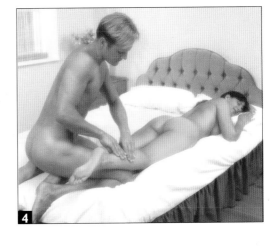

Remember to add oil whenever your hands start rasping as they cross skin.

But no one said you had to add it with your hands. Try smoothing it onto any part of your body and rubbing against your partner to share it.

1. As you rub some more oil in, take time to enjoy the feeling of your lover's skin, smooth, warm and glistening.

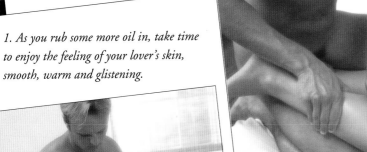

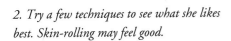

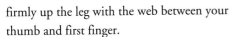

2. Try a few techniques to see what she likes best. Skin-rolling may feel good.

3. Give a long firm rub with the web between your finger and thumb.

6. Erotic massage is about enjoying the feel of each other in every way.

4. Speed up a little with a series of quick squeezes all the way up her calf muscle.

5. You don't have to lie down – why not experiment with different positions?

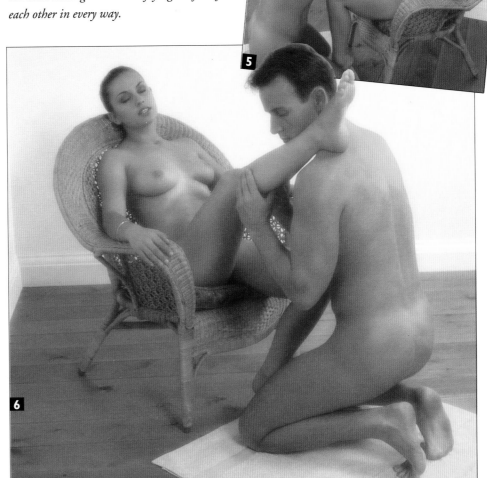

firmly up the leg with the web between your thumb and first finger.

Continue by ***hacking*** briskly with the sides of your hands, ***tapping*** with fingertips or ***drumming*** with loose fists up and down the calf muscle – check you're not doing this too hard. Finish off with a few long, slow, soothing ***strokes*** up to the knee.

You can use all these techniques once or twice each, or just one repeated several times – whatever your partner likes best and you like doing. Throughout the massage you can experiment, stick to your favourites or try all of them, as long as you generally start and end with stroking moves.

Thighs & Buttocks

Most couples find that a sensual massage of the buttocks is a highly arousing and erotic experience, particularly if it is carried out in an intimately lit and comfortable setting. Take your time to build up the feelings of pleasure.

Stroke gently over the back of the knee then, with more pressure, up over the thigh and buttock. You'll need to spread your hands out more than on the calf as you bring them back, running your hands down both sides of the thigh. If you feel you're leaning too far, move forward and kneel astride the calf, being careful not to put your weight on it.

The best moves on the thigh and up over the buttock are **kneading**, **thumb-rolling** and **rubbing**. When kneading, work on the outside of the thigh as well as the top, and all over the buttock.

Follow this by **hacking** or **drumming** all over the thigh and buttock. Spreading one hand over the buttock and **shaking** it firmly can feel good too.

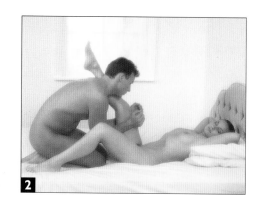

2. There aren't any set rules – if she's more relaxed lying on her back, go with it.

3. Add some more oil as you work on this delicate part of her body.

1. Use your wrists and arms to create a smooth even pressure for a sensation you are both sure to enjoy.

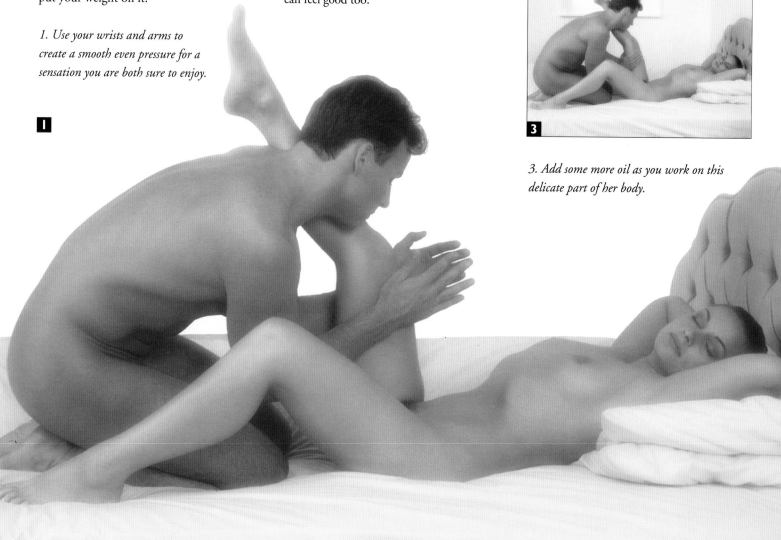

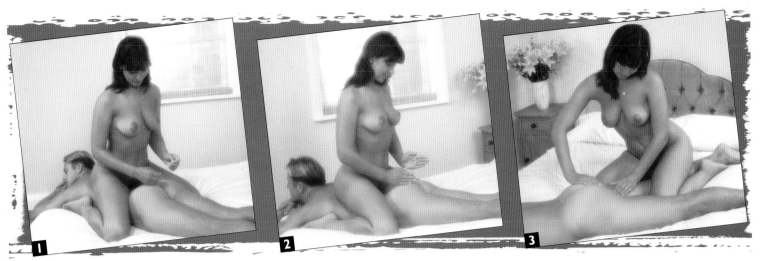

1. *Percussion moves are both relaxing to muscles and stimulating to the skin.*

2. *Hacking feels good here too: just keep it light and well away from the spine.*

3. *Kneading and squeezing and stroking also feel good for both partners.*

Try some **skin-rolling** over the fleshy areas of the thighs and buttocks. Gently lift a handful of flesh in each hand, and bring the fingers back towards the thumbs step by step rather than sliding them across the skin. Let go before your fingers and thumb come close enough to pinch, and work your way over all parts that have enough flesh to lift.

Right: Flesh, muscle and very sensitive skin in this area mean you can hardly go wrong whatever techniques you use.

Below: A sexy grab or a loving, tender touch – anything you do here is likely to give pleasure both to you and to your lover.

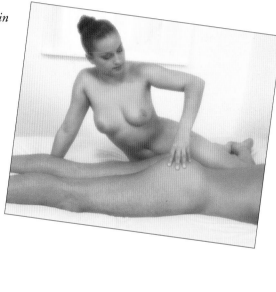

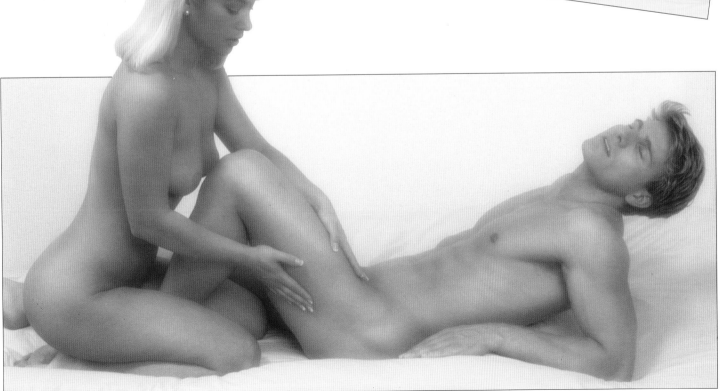

More Thighs & Buttocks

When you're receiving a massage, focus on the pleasure your body is giving you. Don't waste time worrying that your partner is judging your skin tone or body shape. This is a good time for building trust between you.

The thighs and buttocks have large muscles which carry a lot of tension – the legs from carrying the whole body's weight and the buttocks from keeping the back upright – so deep muscle work like kneading helps unknot them. But be kind; this can be quite painful.

The layers of flesh we tend to carry in these areas can benefit too, from moves like *plucking* which improve the blood circulation. Taking little handfuls of flesh, pluck lightly all over the buttocks and the outside of the thighs.

Hacking, *tapping*, *drumming* and *cupping* work well here too. Remember to keep your wrists loose and your shoulders relaxed: you're aiming to stimulate and excite, not to jolt or hurt.

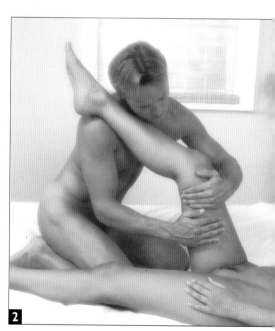

1. Vary the pressure from light to firm, always going up towards her body.

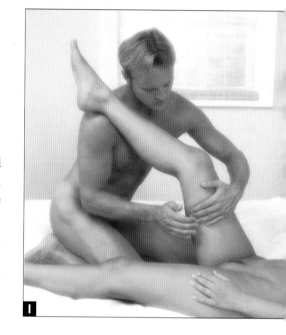

2. Try to keep the movements continuous in a silky, well-oiled rhythm.

3. Most people enjoy the feeling of their lover stroking their thighs.

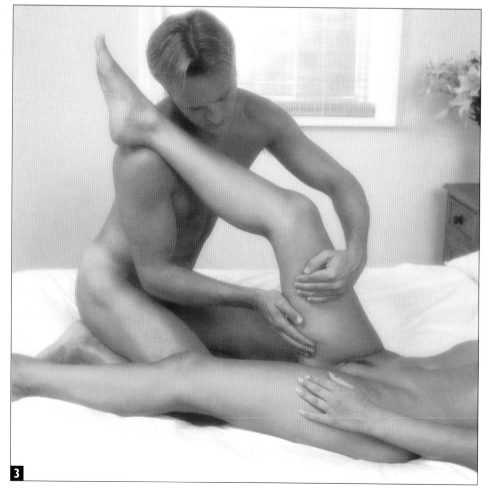

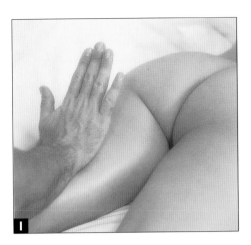

1. Hand pressure may feel good around the thigh and buttocks.

This is a sexy, enjoyable area to massage, whether you're giving or receiving it. Squeezing, stroking and kneading come naturally. In fact almost anything you do here will feel good, for both of you.

Explore with fingernails, tongue — even little slaps or nips with your teeth. This is the likeliest point for a massage to take a delightful detour into sweaty, rolling, all-in wrestling sex.

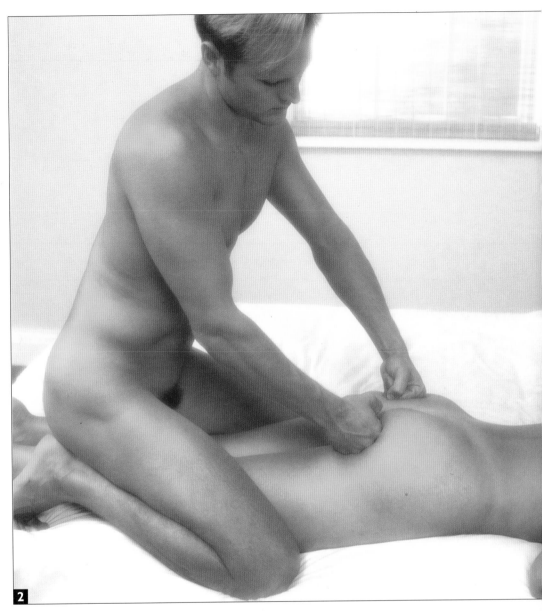

2. As well as being a sexy spot, this holds a surprising amount of muscle tension.

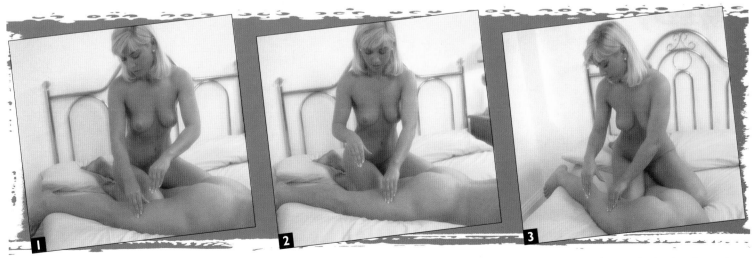

1. Try some of the lightest, most arousing movements on his thighs.

2. Start plucking his skin, working up and down and around the thigh.

3. Change to 'picking up feathers' and note the different sensations.

Shoulders

If you've resisted the temptation to forget about techniques and dive on top of your lover – or if you've enjoyed that intermission and you're ready for more – the massage journey continues further up.

Give someone a really effective back and shoulder massage and they'll be putty in your hands. Women have said yes to outrageous propositions at this point. Men have been known to agree they'll go to the ballet.

Run your hands smoothly in one long *stroke* from the buttocks up beside the spine to the neck and rest your hands on your partner's shoulders for a while, tapping into that feeling of closeness you created at the beginning. For this area, it's best if he rests his forehead, face-down, on a rolled-up towel or on his forearms rather than lying with head to one side.

You can work on this area while kneeling beside your lover, sitting astride his back or kneeling in front of him, his head resting between your thighs. If you work from one side, don't forget to swap and do the other.

Experiment with different positions and moves to find the most effective combination. This area holds so much everyday tension that he will really appreciate a massage that gets to grips with

1. For most of us, shoulders hold more tension than any other part of our bodies.

2. Having these tight muscles unknotted puts you in a relaxed and tender mood.

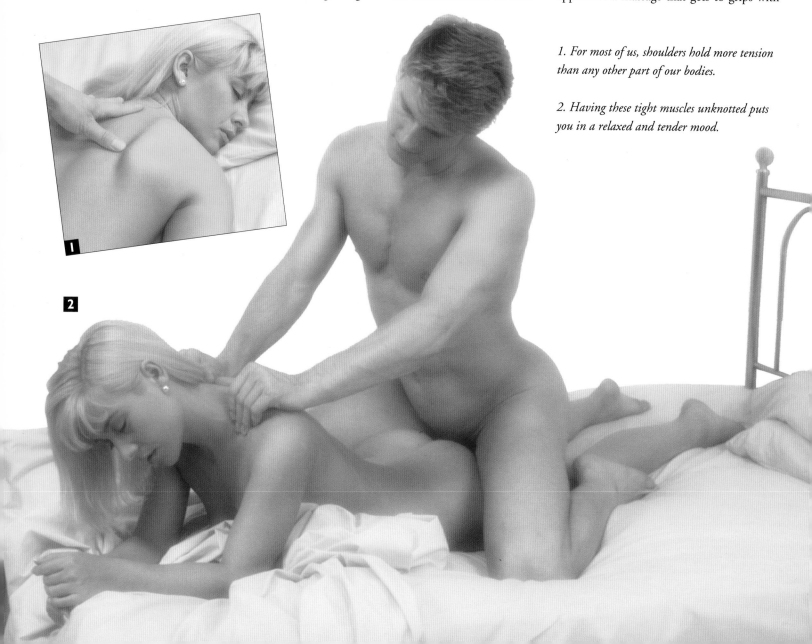

1

2

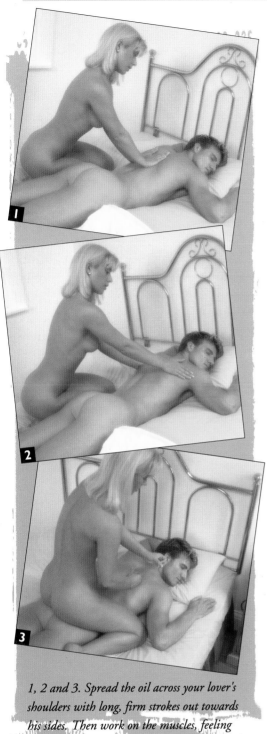

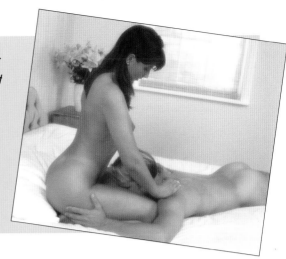

If he's lying with his head between your thighs his arms are likely to have slipped around you and his tongue may be dreamily exploring your warmth.

Continue stroking rhythmically down his neck and back and just go with the flow.

1, 2 and 3. Spread the oil across your lover's shoulders with long, firm strokes out towards his sides. Then work on the muscles, feeling them start to loosen up under your fingers.

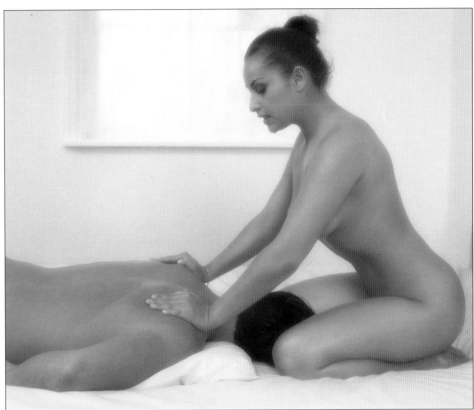

Finish with some long, slow, soothing strokes and stay for a while with your hands still on his back, enhancing the feeling of peace and connectedness between you.

his muscles. Kneading and deep stroking moves do the most good here.

Start by *stroking* quite firmly over the whole shoulder area, outwards from the neck and down the spine. Then *knead* the big muscles over the top of the shoulders with both hands. If he's not too sensitive you can work with both hands on one shoulder, kneading and *skin-rolling* – holding a handful of muscle and walking the fingers towards the thumb. This is particularly helpful on well developed muscles.

Thumb-rolling up or down the spine will feel good too, sliding the thumbs firmly along beside the spine one at a time, each one starting to move just before you lift the other. Don't forget to include some *hand pressure* in slow circling movements over the whole muscular area at the top of the back. If you're kneeling beside him or sitting on him, slip your hands down over the shoulders, hold them firmly so your hands don't slip and give a gentle *stretch* by pulling slowly backwards.

Alternate reverse stroking is a lovely soothing way to end, especially if you've done some quite deep work. Finish with some long, slow, firm stroking movements over the whole area and rest again for a while with your hands on his shoulders.

Neck & Head from the Back

Lift your partner's hair off her neck and spread it over the top of her head, leaving her ears visible. You may need to comb your fingers through it to stop it falling back, but this has a pleasing feel of its own.

For this part of the massage, you'll need to be either beside your partner or kneeling astride her back, since you want to work up the top of the spine. The general rule of massage is to assist the blood circulation by working towards the heart, which in this case would be down the spine – but try it and you'll find it just doesn't work.

Starting between the shoulder blades, massage up beside the spine with a firm *thumb-rolling* motion, making sure you have enough oil on your hands.

Support your partner's forehead with one hand, **grip** the back of her neck with the other and pull fingers and thumb towards each other without letting them slide over

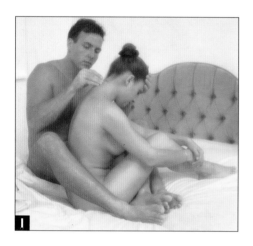

1. *Support her forehead safely with your hand.*

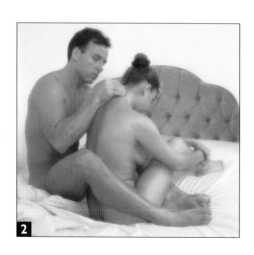

2. *Hair needs to be kept out of the way for this.*

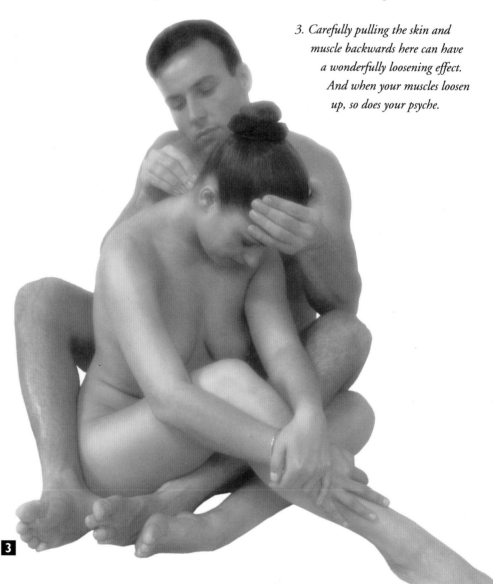

3. *Carefully pulling the skin and muscle backwards here can have a wonderfully loosening effect. And when your muscles loosen up, so does your psyche.*

her skin. Stop short of pinching, and repeat slowly several times.

When you reach the base of the skull, spread your fingers out over the scalp and massage along under the edge of the skull from beside the ears towards the spine with **thumb circles.**

With hands pressed firmly on each side of her scalp, try to **push your hands towards each other** as if your fingertips would meet at the top of her head. The idea is to move the scalp over the skull, not to let the fingers slip across the scalp and pull her hair. You need a finely judged pressure here to avoid pulling her hair without putting a vicelike grip on her head, but it's worth getting it right. We don't think of the head as a place that holds tension but it does – as every good hairdresser knows when she throws in a few minutes' head massage – and this helps release it.

Finish this part of the massage by holding your lover's head safely between your hands for a few moments, then ask her to turn onto her back.

3. The way we live and work constantly overstresses our neck and shoulder muscles.

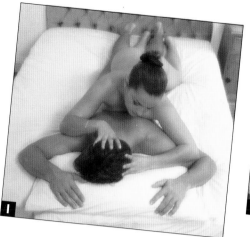

1. Clasp his head and push your fingertips towards each other, trying to move his scalp.

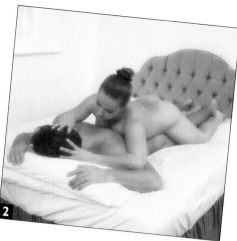

2. Aim to make the skin slide slightly, without pulling the hair or pressing into the head.

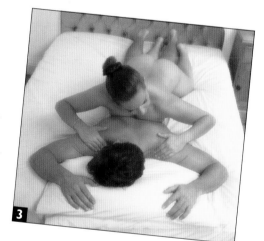

This is a good time to stop and enjoy the intimacy of the mood you are creating.

❧

Lie beside or on top of your lover, close together, and both stretch out to the ends of your fingers and toes.

❧

Bring your fingertips and toes back along his limbs with the lightest, spine-tingling touch.

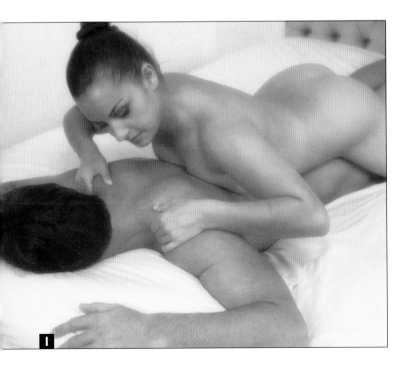

1. It's surprising how tight both the skin and the muscles feel here.

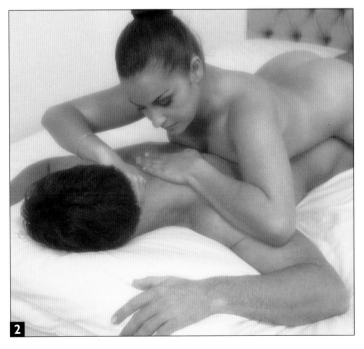

2. The neck is a vulnerable area, so keep all your moves slow and gentle.

Feet

Start work on the front of your lover's body by kneeling holding his feet for a moment. A foot massage is the perfect moment to appreciate the wonderful structure of the human body, which we take so easily for granted.

The 26 fine bones in each foot adapt to every step on unnatural man-made surfaces with rarely a complaint. Now's the time to give our overworked, maltreated feet the tender loving care they deserve.

You may need to adjust your touch here to strike the right balance. 'Gentle' is the word to keep in mind – there's very little flesh to cushion the complex and delicate bone structure – but don't go so lightly that it tickles. Support your lover's knee with a rolled-up towel if he finds it uncomfortable when you hold his foot up.

Put one of his feet back on the bed or floor and, resting the other one on your lap, *stroke* it from toes to ankle. Next, holding it in both hands, make large *thumb circles* over the whole of the top of the foot.

Grip the outside of the foot with thumbs on the sole and pull fingers and thumbs gently towards each other. Most of the pressure is going from the thumb into the sole.

We hardly ever take the time to pamper our feet – or to realise their erotic potential.

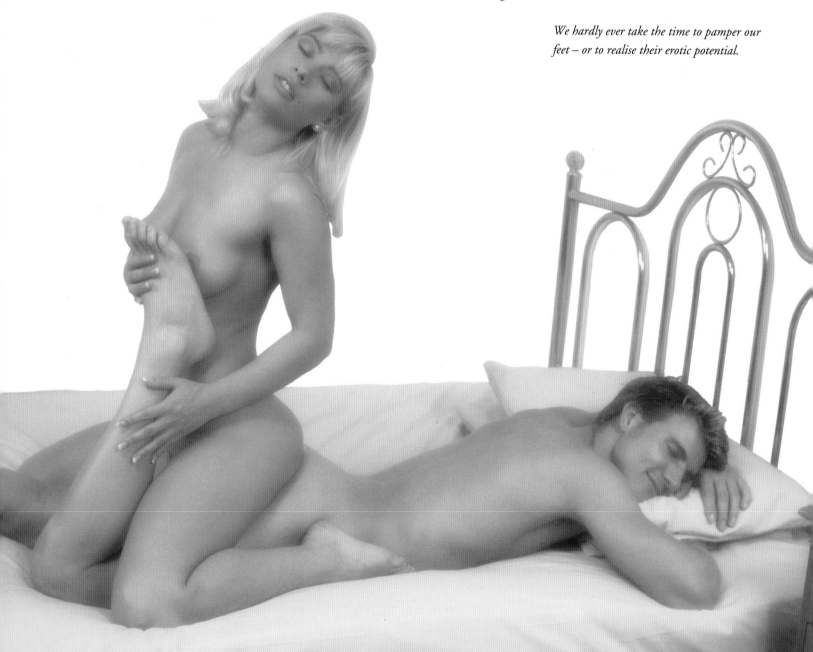

Toes have an even harder time than the rest of the foot, especially women's – high-heeled shoes throw all the weight onto the front of the foot, which wasn't made to carry it alone, and the toes end up squashed. So *pull* and *knead* each toe separately. ***Squeeze*** the pad of each toe and let go quickly. Starting between the toes, ***thumb-roll*** smoothly up (between the bones continuing up from the toes) towards the ankle.

Knuckle the sole of the foot, ***thumb-roll*** from heel to toes and make ***thumb circles*** all over the sole. Always hold the foot securely so your lover can fully relax.

Repeat the whole sequence with the other foot, and take some time doing whatever your partner most likes. Feet rarely get a chance like this.

1. Hold the foot just firmly enough not to tickle, without putting pressure on these small bones.

2. Run your thumbs towards the ankle, between the bones extending from the toes.

It's odd how sexy feet are. Despite the hard work and abuse they endure, they're full of exciting little nerve endings that thrill to the right kind of touch.

For many people, a foot massage is better than any other kind. So if your partner is blissing out while you knead his feet, stay with it.

Run your fingertips lightly down to his toes and the backs of your fingernails up to his ankles. Nibble his toes, pulling them slightly with your teeth, and run your tongue lightly around his ankle bones.

If he's not ticklish, and he's just come out of the bath, try running your tongue over the soles of his feet.

3. Cover the top of the foot with large, light thumb circles and stroke towards the ankles.

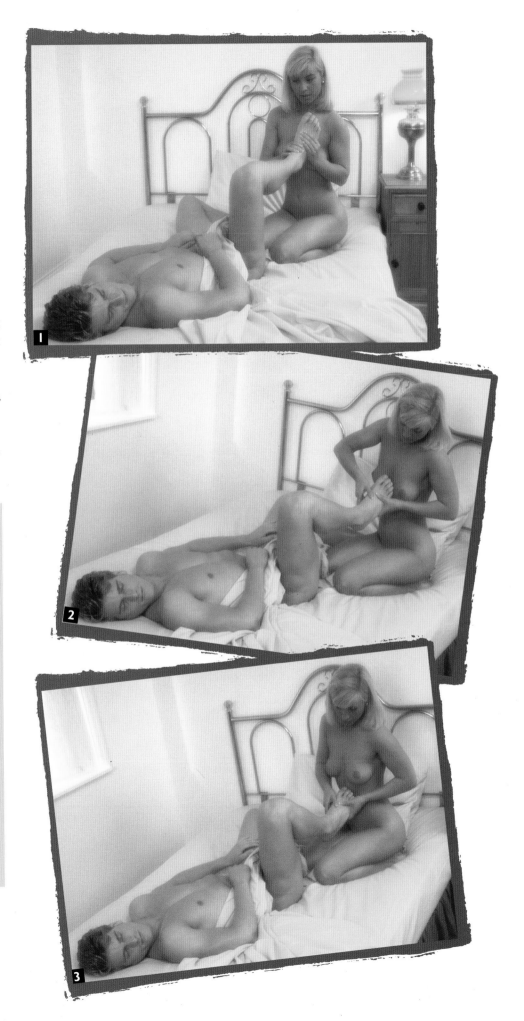

Front of the Legs

Even someone as close to you as your lover may feel uncomfortably exposed lying naked on her back when you're not making love. Don't feel rejected — she's probably worrying how she looks, or feeling strangely defenceless.

Most of us rarely give our bodies a thought except to criticize our (often imaginary) flaws. Even sex can be a brief and localized thrill, leaving most of our capacity for pleasure untapped. We mainly live in our heads, or maybe our stomachs or genitals. Massage helps bring us back into our whole bodies, fully occupying them

Stroke up into your lover's groin and fan your hands up over the hipbones. Repeat this several times, letting your thumbs brush past the pubic hair.

❧

For a woman, gradually let your thumbs slide lightly between her lips as you continue the stroking movement. Add some oil if necessary so they glide smoothly through.

For a man, let your thumbs outline his genitals on the way past with a teasingly light touch. Don't worry, you'll be back.

1. With fingers pointing inwards, stroke firmly up with one hand then the other.

2. This is a moment to massage gently, while appreciating the beauty of your lover's body.

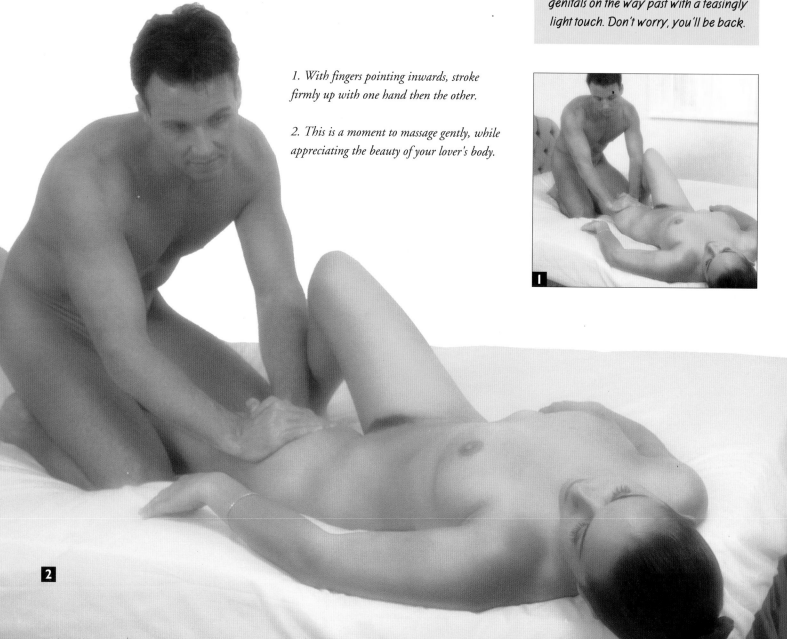

1

2

down to our toes and hairtips, out to every inch of skin and including the parts we don't care much about – like the body's natural curves. This is a time to celebrate and enjoy them all.

Start with a long firm *stroke* up the front of the leg from ankle to upper thigh, using both hands. Fan out at the top and come back lightly down the sides of the leg. Do the same but stroking up the sides of the legs and bringing your hands as far round to the back as they'll go.

Below the knee is mainly bone, so you won't be doing much work on it. If there's enough muscle beside it, you can gently knead up both sides of the shin with little *thumb circles*. Finish by *stroking* upwards, or with one stroke down a hairy leg to stop it feeling prickly – making sure you have enough oil to avoid pulling the hair.

Massage the knee by slipping both hands underneath, fingers pointing down, and pulling them gently towards the front to give a feeling of opening. Put one hand on the near side of the thigh, fingers pointing up, and the other on the far side pointing down. Slide them backwards and

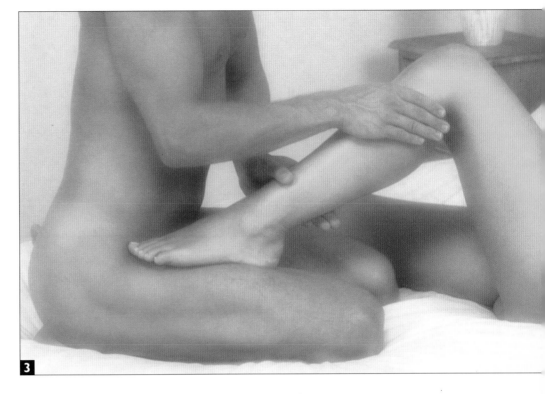

forwards past each other in a *criss-crossing* move, passing each other at the top of the thigh. Work from just above the knee to near the top of the thigh. Some *thumb-rolling*, *kneading*, *squeezing*, *cupping* or *plucking* may feel good here too.

3. Make a series of thumb circles up beside the bone if you can feel a band of muscle there.

4. On most people there's not much to work on here. Just smooth in the oil with long strokes.

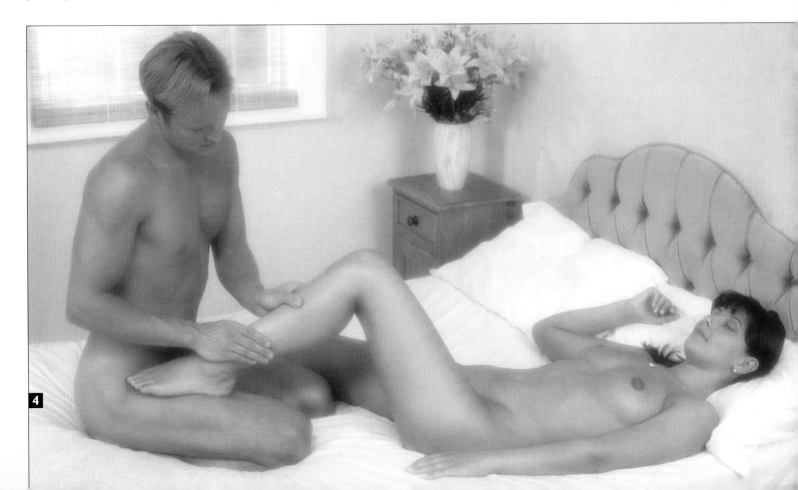

Head & Face

Now change positions to kneel behind your partner's head.
Rest his head on your lap or between your knees, whichever
you both find most comfortable.

Holding the sides of his neck firmly with fingers pointing away from you, pull them firmly back towards yourself, lightening the pressure to let your fingers slip through his hair.

Wipe some oil off your hands before putting them into his hair. Then cup his head in your hands and push them towards the top of his head, making the scalp move slightly over the skull. Or press and make small circles with the palms.

Carefully using fingertips instead of nails, lightly 'scratch' all over his head. Keeping your thumbs still, as an anchor, **knead** the scalp in small circles with the fingertips. Run your fingers through his hair and gently fan it outwards as you continue the movement.

Support your partner's
head comfortably so your
movements don't push it
from side to side.

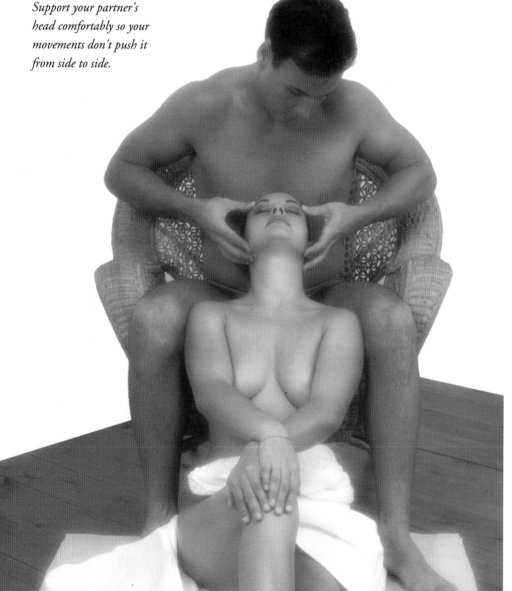

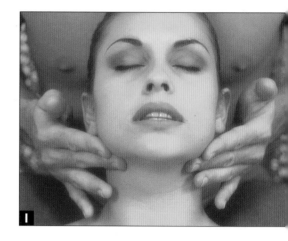

1. Lightly stroke up from the collar bones.

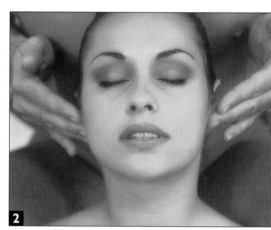

2. Always stroke upwards and outwards.

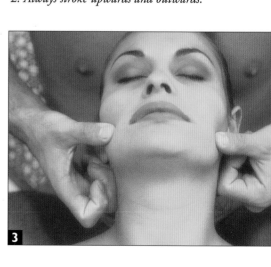

3. Trace the edges of the jaw with thumb circles.

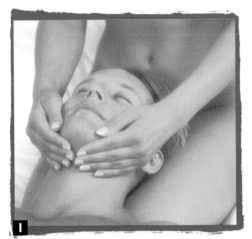

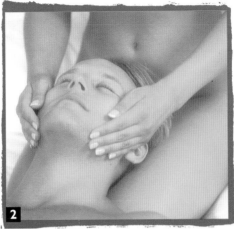

1.Keep your hands still for a few moments.

2. The warmth of your hands is relaxing in itself.

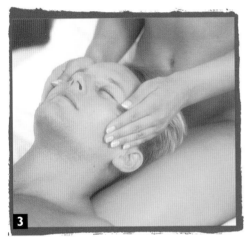

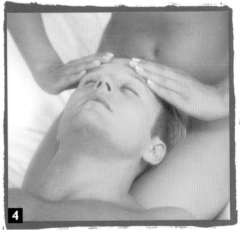

3. Make skin gently slide, as you did on the scalp.

4. This can ease headaches or even prevent them.

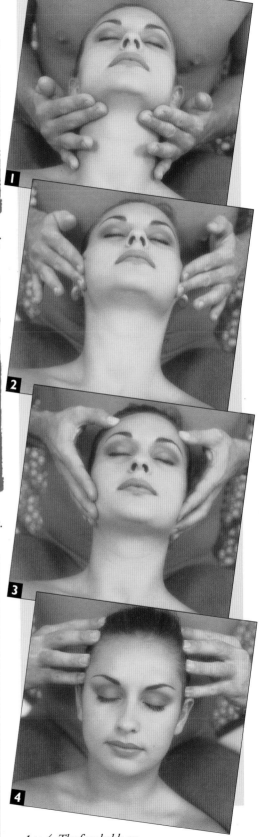

Add more oil and smooth it into his face and neck, keeping a safe distance from the eyes. Massage it in with long strokes of your fingerpads, upwards and outwards. Follow his jawline, cheekbones, around the mouth, up the temples and across the forehead. Anywhere you feel tightness – because the face holds a lot of tension, especially around the jaw – massage with little *finger* and *thumb circles*.

Using firm pressure, put your thumbs one each side of the bridge of his nose and *stroke* out along his eyebrows. Repeat a fraction higher up and continue until you're stroking along the hairline. For a change, you could also stroke from the centre of his forehead to the temples with alternating thumbs. Then *tap* all over the face with your fingertips or pads.

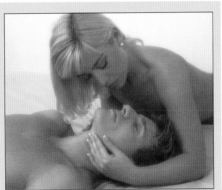

Lightly trace the contours of his face with your fingertips, moving upwards with a featherlight touch. You could follow this with a trail of kisses.

Finish by holding his face cupped in your hands for a few moments.

1 to 4. The face holds an extraordinary amount of daily tension and responds blissfully to being gently massaged. This also helps smooth out first signs of wrinkles.

Chest & Breasts

Sliding your hands down from the face, press your partner's shoulders firmly away from you, towards her feet. Then run your hands onto her chest and spread the oil around with broad, circular strokes.

With palms flat and fingertips facing away from you, **reverse stroke** firmly up beside the breastbone with both hands at once. Do the same around the outside of the breasts, but don't put direct pressure on the nipples. Then use your fingertips to circle and spiral around the breasts in either direction.

Vary this with light pressure and featherlight touch, but always start near the nipple and finish at the armpit. Continue the stroke up into the armpit if your partner doesn't find this ticklish – it can be a surprisingly erogenous zone. Massaging the muscles between the ribs, close to the breastbone, with **thumb circles** may also feel good.

Women may find their breasts change in sensitivity during the month, so that what they enjoy at one time may become painful just before a period is due. In this case, you could try some reflexology instead. Do some **thumb-rolling** up the top of her feet, covering a couple of inches from the base of the toes. Working on this spot is said to ease sore breasts.

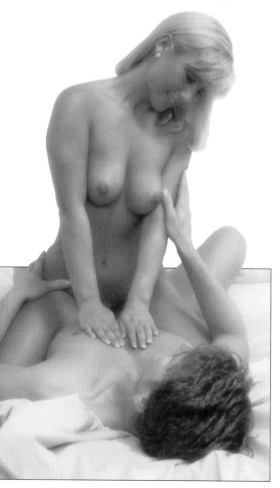

Above: Whenever you're giving a massage, keep experimenting to discover things that feel even better for you and your partner.

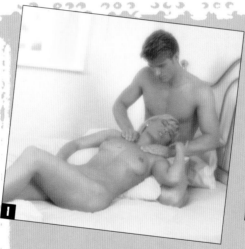

1. Vary your touch from light to barely there.

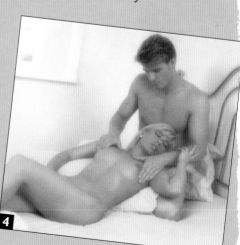

2. Stroke between the ribs from the breast

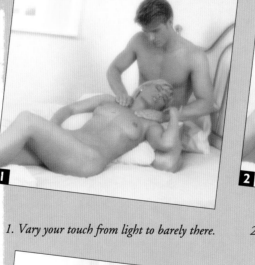

3. Spiral delicately outwards from the nipples.

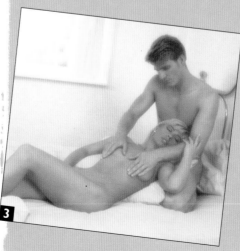

4. Be aware of times when her breasts are

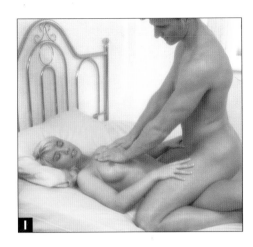

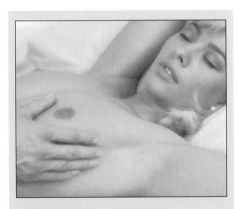

1. A long, firm stroke upwards between the breasts and out towards the shoulders across the upper chest gives a lifting, opening feeling that most people like.

2 and 3. Take time to play and explore – find out how toes feel on ribs and nipples on soles.

Nipples are the most overtly sexy part of the body. But people vary in the way they like them touched. Some enjoy a lot of stroking, squeezing, sucking and even nibbling. Others like very gentle treatment, such as a dream touch spiralling from the nipples out to the armpits, or very light flicking with the tongue.

How much you play with your lover's breasts depends entirely on how sensual she (or he) finds this. But practically everyone enjoys a caressing stroke upward and outward.

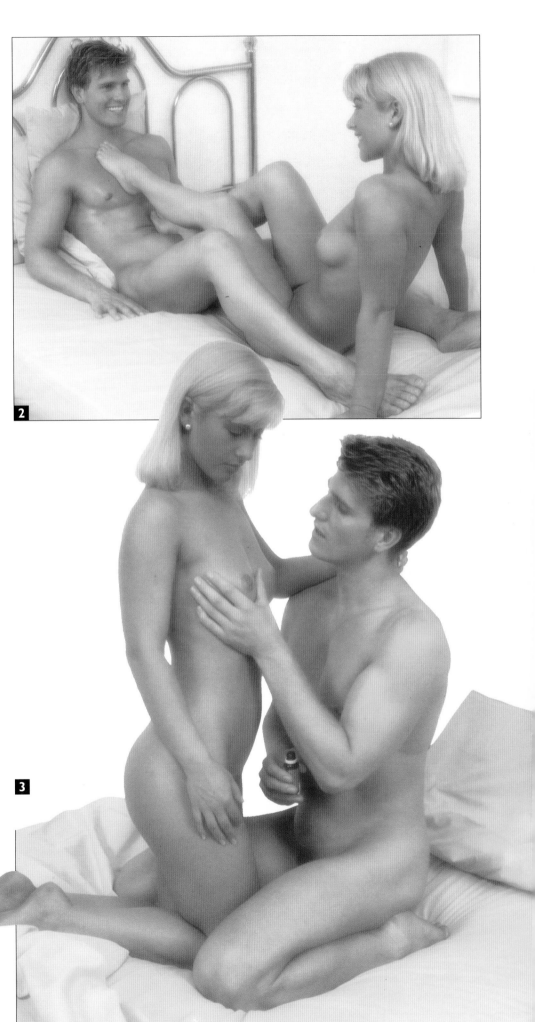

Hands & Arms

Kneel beside your partner and hold one of her hands in both of yours for a few moments. Lift the arm to give it a gentle stretch before putting it back on the bed.

Now *knead* her palm and the fleshy area round the base of the thumb with your thumbs. Knead each finger, then hold it tight and pull up to the tip as if pulling a glove off. *Stroke* firmly up the back of the hand with your palm and run your thumb up from between the fingers.

Interlace your fingers with hers and gently bend them back to stretch her palm. Then hold her hand and push it back and forth and round in a circle to flex the wrist.

Rest her arm on the bed and start *cross-stroking*. Put your hands on her forearm, your right hand pointing left above your left

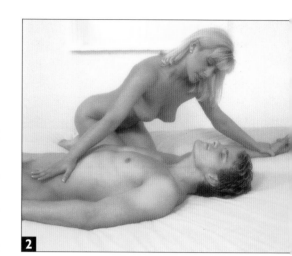

2

1. Raise your lover's arm, telling him to let you take all the weight, then move it in a circle to give a feeling of movement and openness.

2. Next, stretch the arm out gently to the side and give it a light shake to help release tension before putting it carefully back down.

hand pointing right. Stroke firmly up with the right hand, doing the same with the left one as you lift away your right hand. Work your way up her arm with alternating strokes.

Put your hand around her wrist, *squeeze* and release. Work your way up the arm squeezing and releasing, then go down to the elbow and work up from there doing the same from under the arm. Run your hand up her arm, *rubbing* with the skin between your thumb and first finger. *Kneading*, *plucking*, *hand pressure*, *cupping* and *criss-crossing* can all feel good on muscular arms.

Finally, hold her hand in one of yours and *stroke* firmly all the way up her arm with the other, taking the movement right over her shoulder and pulling the shoulder downwards before bringing your hand back down the underside of her arm. Repeat several times. Then step over to her other side and do the same for the other hand and arm.

Right: Women tend to have a lot less noticeable muscle in their arms than men, so they're likely to prefer the delicate techniques here, such as stroking, gentle squeezing and light plucking.

If she's dying to join in by this time, she may not let go of your hand.

≈

Try some dual massage: entwined in each other's arms and legs, massage each other with every movable part — your chin against her shoulder, her heels kneading your buttocks, your bellies pressing each other with each in-breath.

1. Don't forget the hands, too. Squeeze the sides, thumb-circle the palm and slide your fist down each finger as if pulling tight gloves off.

2. Unlike most of the body, hands feel good massaged in either direction: either up towards the wrist or down to the fingertips.

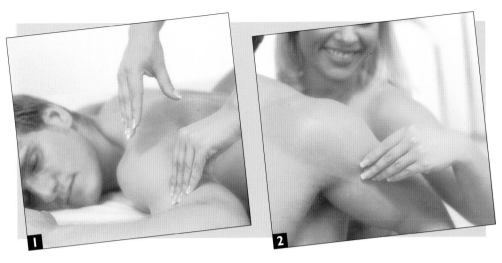

1. Work up his arms, kneading and gripping.   *2. These strong moves feel good on large muscles.*

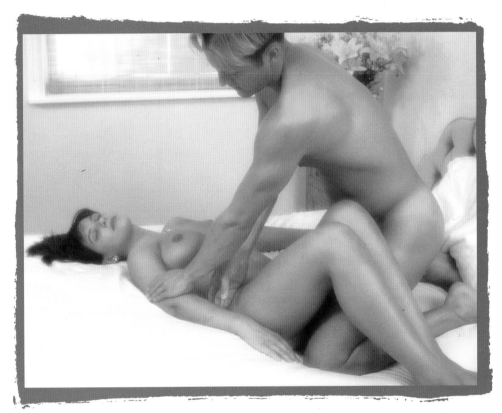

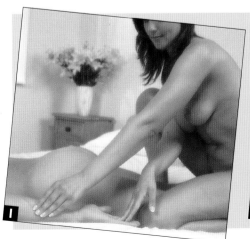
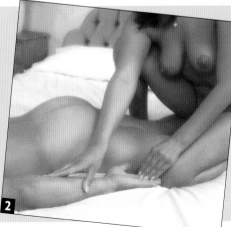

The Abdomen

There's a lot happening here, and the right touch can make this one of the sexiest parts of the body.

Most people feel slightly vulnerable when anyone touches their stomach, even in the safe atmosphere of a loving massage. This is natural, since this area contains so many vital organs that are easy to hurt. But that same sensitivity makes this a highly erogenous zone. Oriental traditions hold that you can arouse the body's vital energies by massaging the abdomen.

It's also the one part of their own body that both men and women tend to dislike. So if your lover, no matter how slim or toned, is feeling like a blob, this is the moment to show your appreciation of that sexy flesh.

Slow, sensuous *stroking* moves feel good here. Start with your hands under his waist, fingertips pointing towards each other, and slightly lift his back.

Then pull your hands firmly towards the front, turning as as they come onto his stomach to point downwards. Complete the move by stroking down towards his pubic bone, circling out to the sides and back to the starting point.

Thumb-roll downwards from the navel, then work your way down from the navel with *thumb pressure*, moving about a fingerwidth at a time.

When you reach the pubic area, make sure your hands are well oiled and change to slow stroking movements, including the perineum – the stretch of skin just behind the genitals in both sexes. Vary the pressure from quite firm, especially for a man, to tantalizingly light.

The testicles and clitoris are, of course, highly sensitive, so while direct pressure is painful, a firm stroking movement around the sides followed by a featherlight stroke is exquisitely sensual. In this area more than ever, listen to what your partner likes and notice how her body responds – whether she's melting with pleasure or tensing up uncomfortably.

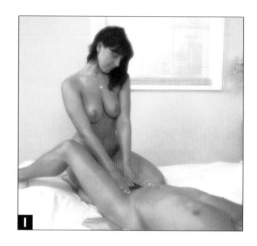

1. Imagine a line drawn from his navel, then work your way down it with thumb pressure.

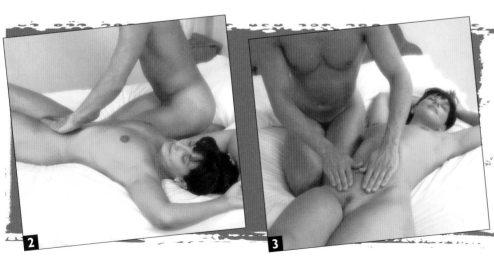

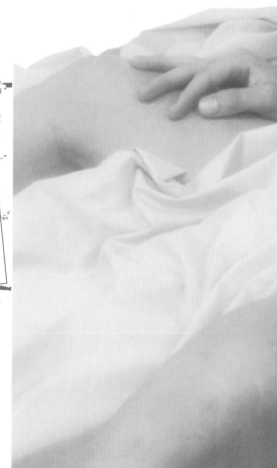

2. Using firm pressure, bring your hands up from under her waist to meet beside her navel. Then continue down her abdomen in one long flowing movement, with lighter pressure.

3. Thumb-roll slowly downwards from the navel with well-oiled hands. Here you can either pause for a moment with your hands on her abdomen, or slide down towards her thighs.

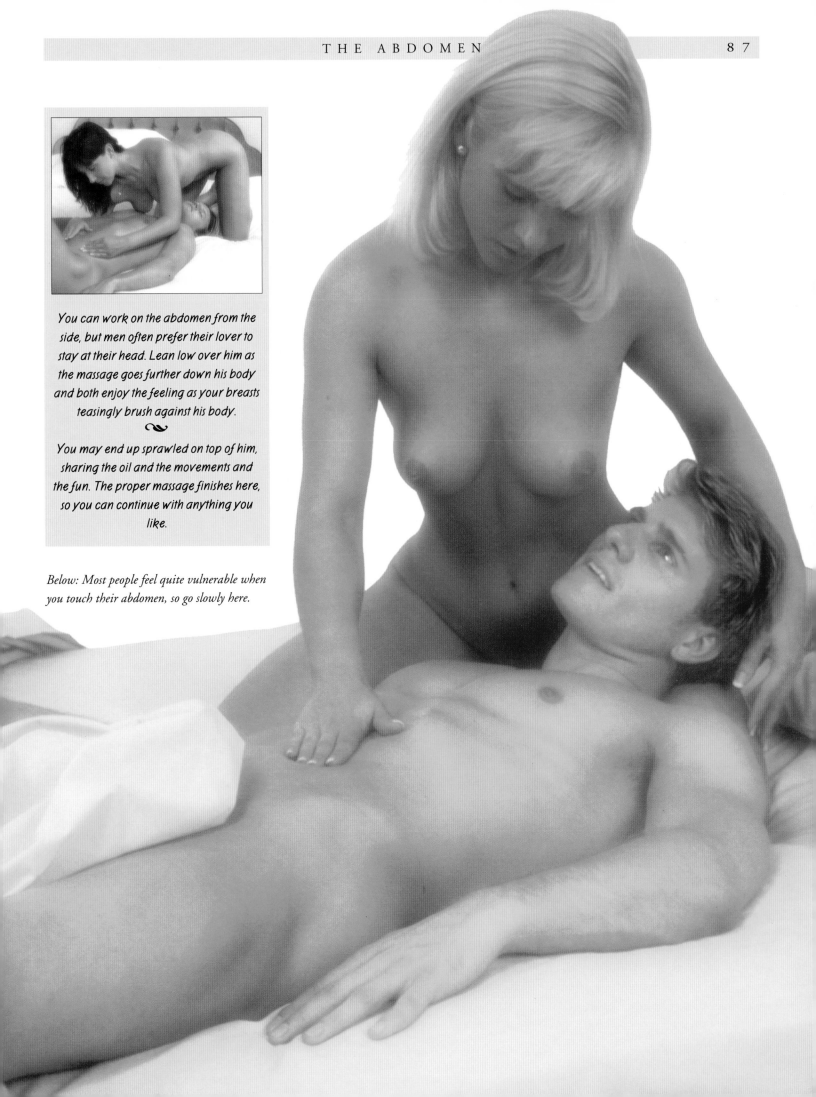

You can work on the abdomen from the side, but men often prefer their lover to stay at their head. Lean low over him as the massage goes further down his body and both enjoy the feeling as your breasts teasingly brush against his body.

❧

You may end up sprawled on top of him, sharing the oil and the movements and the fun. The proper massage finishes here, so you can continue with anything you like.

Below: Most people feel quite vulnerable when you touch their abdomen, so go slowly here.

Massage in Pregnancy

Pregnancy gives women a beauty bonus; silky hair, glowing skin and voluptuous breasts for even the skinniest. Women are often at their sexiest and most vibrant during pregnancy.

Many pregnant women may have times of feeling ugly and clumsy. Changing hormone levels affect their moods, and the irritations of pregnancy – backache, constipation and swollen ankles – can leave a woman feeling more burdened than blessed.

Massage goes a long way towards solving all these problems, not least in helping the woman remember she has a whole body to enjoy. Even if she's not in the mood for passion, she'll still appreciate a rub for her aching feet and back. Just check with the doctor that there's no reason not to. An arm massage can be wonderfully relaxing if other areas of the body feel too uncomfortable to touch, and upper-back massage may relieve morning sickness.

Pregnancy can be a highly erotic time, with no worries about contraception, while a surge of feminine hormones makes a woman more attractive than ever. If ordinary sex becomes uncomfortable during the later months, massage offers imaginative variations that won't cause any physical strain.

Obviously as the baby grows she won't want to lie on her front, and lying on her back may leave her feeling like a beached whale. The most comfortable positions are lying on her side, with her upper leg bent and supported by pillows, or sitting astride a chair with some cushions for padding.

Essential oils are strong enough to be used for medical purposes, so they can have powerful effects. Pregnant women shouldn't either give or receive massage with oils of cedarwood, clary sage, cypress, jasmine, juniper, marjoram, myrrh or valerian. (That's just from the oils mentioned in this book – check separately if you want to use any others.) In the first three months of pregnancy they should also avoid camomile, geranium, lavender and rose.

Strangely enough, ankle massage may possibly cause miscarriage, so keep away from this area when giving a relaxing foot rub.

Right: Use unscented oil if she's suffering from nausea. From the fifth month onwards you can safely massage her abdomen and lower back.

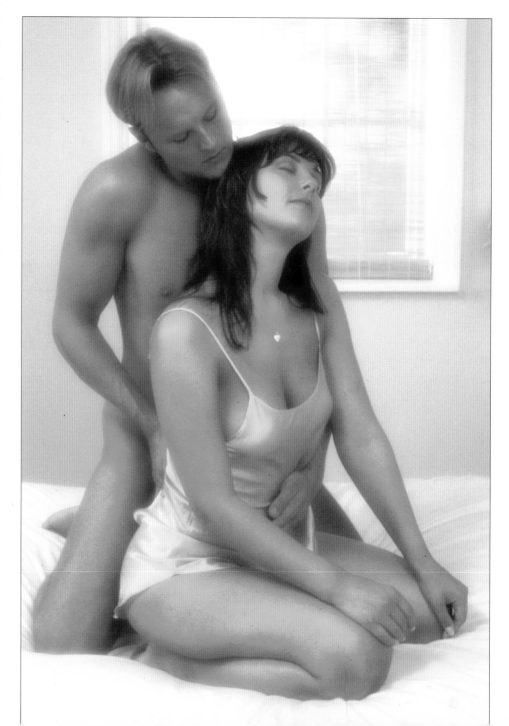

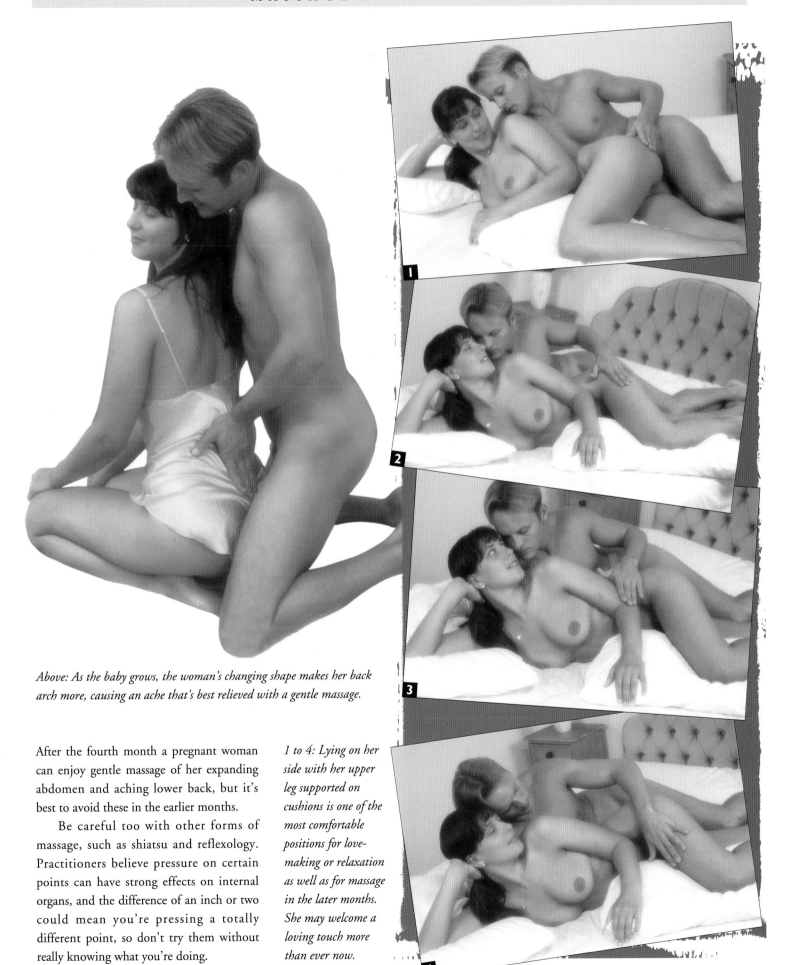

Above: As the baby grows, the woman's changing shape makes her back arch more, causing an ache that's best relieved with a gentle massage.

After the fourth month a pregnant woman can enjoy gentle massage of her expanding abdomen and aching lower back, but it's best to avoid these in the earlier months.

Be careful too with other forms of massage, such as shiatsu and reflexology. Practitioners believe pressure on certain points can have strong effects on internal organs, and the difference of an inch or two could mean you're pressing a totally different point, so don't try them without really knowing what you're doing.

1 to 4: Lying on her side with her upper leg supported on cushions is one of the most comfortable positions for love-making or relaxation as well as for massage in the later months. She may welcome a loving touch more than ever now.

Shiatsu

If you're feeling adventurous, why not try an oriental technique that aims to stimulate the body's flow of energy? Its movements, totally different from western massage, can give an invigorating shot of vitality. If you hit the right spot, you may be awakening passionate energies you hadn't dreamed of. Ready to be recharged?

nstead of rubbing or kneading, shiatsu practitioners press straight in with the tips of their thumbs. This Japanese form of massage, known in

a slightly different Chinese version as acupressure, works on a series of precise spots all over the body. According to oriental medical tradition, vital energy circulates in a network of 'meridians' criss-crossing the entire body like a road map, just as the veins and arteries carry blood. Pressing on different spots along these meridians is said to tone up or calm down the body's energies and even work on the internal organs. As you massage your way round your partner's body, you could try a few shiatsu points, keeping up the pressure for about 10 seconds.

Sexual energy stems from a point in the abdomen that, according to this tradition, is the centre of the body. To find it, put your partner's hand across her abdomen with the index finger just below the navel. Then

Below: You need your lover's help to find the hara, the central point of her body and, according to oriental tradition, the source of sexual energy.

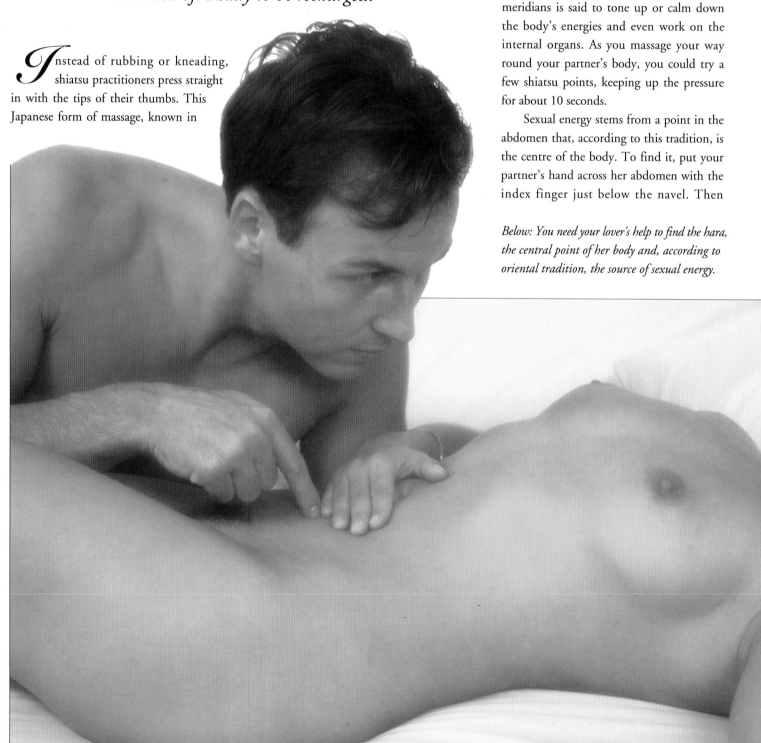

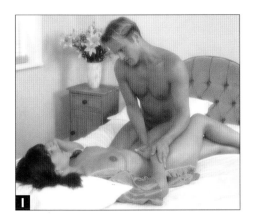

1. Use her hand to measure four fingerwidths.

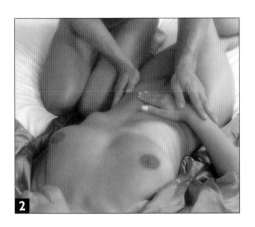

2. Focus your attention on this central spot and imagine energy coursing from it around your body.

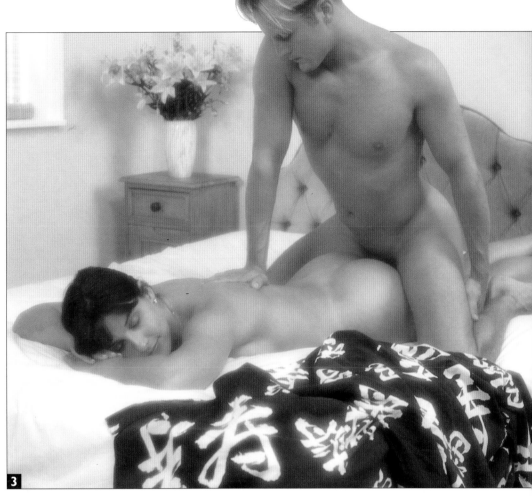

3. To help solve sexual problems, find a point on the spine directly opposite the navel, start by pressing into the muscles beside it and work outwards for about three inches each side.

press the central point below her little finger – in other words, the spot four fingerwidths below the navel. (People have to measure with their own fingers, as someone else's larger or smaller hand would give a wrong measurement.) Pressure here is said to strengthen the body's vital energy – and to arouse desire.

For a shot of stimulating energy, try pinching the front top joint of your partner's little finger, right on the joint. Also, press the centre of her palm or the central crease in the ball of the foot.

Stress and headaches can put a dampener on anyone's ardour – combat them by pressing the point directly between the eyebrows.

And if a night of wild love-making isn't enough to send you to sleep, pinching the earlobes is said to ease insomnia.

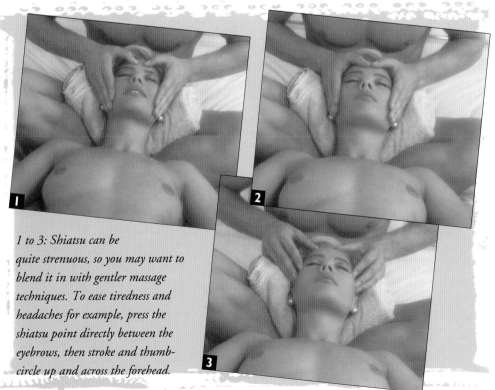

1 to 3: Shiatsu can be quite strenuous, so you may want to blend it in with gentler massage techniques. To ease tiredness and headaches for example, press the shiatsu point directly between the eyebrows, then stroke and thumb-circle up and across the forehead.

Reflexology

Reflexology is much more than an invigorating foot massage, if its practitioners are right. They believe each part of the body is represented by a point on the foot, so massaging that part affects the relevant limb or internal organ.

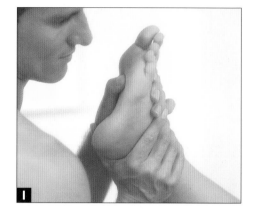

1. For energy, find the solar plexus point, where two sides of the ball of the foot seem to meet.

Reflexology practitioners have 'maps' of the feet, showing how it all fits together – the spine for example, runs up the inner edge of the foot while the big toe represents the head and brain. To give it a try, hold your partner's foot firmly, and press the spot with your thumbs either directly or in small upward strokes.

Sexual arousal

Give your lover an inner buzz by working on the spot halfway between the bottom of each ankle bone and the point of the heel on both sides of each foot (as long as she doesn't wear an IUD). Then massage across the top of the foot from one ankle bone to the other.

Together, all these points represent both men's and women's sex organs, so the massage is meant to tone them up. They can also help with premenstrual syndrome or if either of you loses interest in sex. You could also press the point for the pituitary gland; at the bottom of the big toe pad, right in the middle.

Hangovers

If one of you is feeling off colour after a rich meal or wild party, a spot of reflexology might help your liver cope. Work on the sole about a third of the way between toe and heel of the right foot, running from the third toe to the edge of the foot.

2. If you can't locate a spot directly, you can massage that general area. It's easiest without oil.

Backache

Knead and massage down the inner side of the foot, which represents the spine: the nearer your big toe, the higher up your back.

Aching shoulders

The area across the top and bottom of each foot, about an inch below the toes, represents the shoulders. Since most of us hold some tension there, this is a wonderful area to massage, holding each foot in both hands and pressing in between the bones.

New energy

For when you're feeling too tired for lovemaking. If you run your finger along the ball of your partner's foot, furthest from the toes, you'll find a curve in the middle as if two sections were joined.

This is the solar plexus spot, a very reviving place to massage on either foot. Even better, massage the adrenal point just below in circles with your knuckles at the same time.

Headaches

You can sometimes ease a headache by squeezing the tips of the big toes and the pads just below, which represent the head. This is particularly worth trying as it's said to stimulate the brain too. If it's caused by sinuses, squeeze the sides and back of each toe. To relieve a tired headache across the forehead, press just below the big toenails.

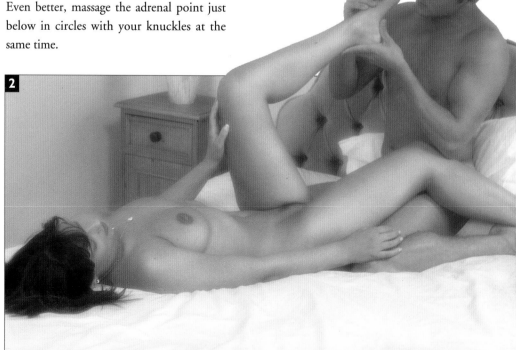

The Head & Shoulder Reviver

Massage isn't just a friendly, loving way to enhance your sex life and increase your capacity for bodily pleasure. A brief neck and shoulder massage can be a life-saver at the end of a stressful day when your lover's too tired to think about having fun. But having the knots eased out of her aching neck may well put her in the mood for more intimate pleasures.

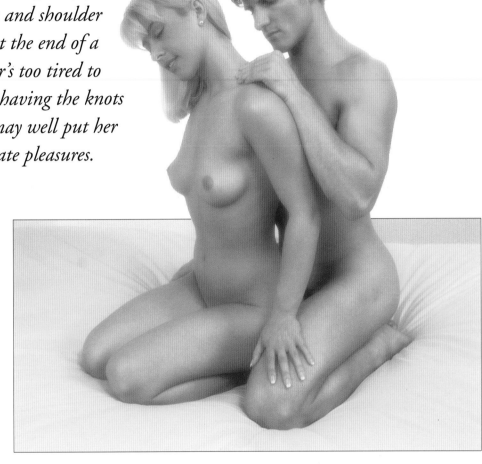

*P*ractically everyone holds tension in their back, neck and shoulders, which makes these the most popular massage spots. Enlightened employers even hire massage therapists to give workers a 10-minute neck and shoulder massage during coffee breaks.

Work with the same smooth, unhurried movements you'd use for a full massage. The one receiving massage should sit astride a chair, leaning on the back with a cushion for padding. You can do the first two moves from either in front or behind, but the rest of the massage works best from the back.

Find the muscular area a couple of inches across from her neck, then put your forearms on her shoulders and **press** down. Too close to the neck it's the wrong bit of muscle and can cause a painful crick, too far away and you're leaning on bone.

Knead the big muscles on top of the shoulders with the heel of your hands and fingers. The mistake people usually make here is digging their fingertips in, which hurts. So keep to the usual massage rule and use the pads of your fingers and thumbs in deep, rhythmic movements. Work across the top of the shoulders and down the upper arms.

Keep one hand on her shoulder to maintain a reassuring contact while you move round behind her if you have been working from in front. Using **hand pressure** across her upper back, make big circles, pressing hard enough to move the underlying muscle without dragging the skin. Avoid direct pressure on the spine.

Grip the back of her neck firmly in one hand and pull fingers and thumb slowly towards the centre. Rest your hands on the back of her head and find the edge of the skull with your thumbs, starting near the bottom of the ears. Massage from the sides across to the centre with both thumbs.

Finish by running your fingers through her hair several times, then settling your hands on her scalp with fingers uppermost. Gently push up as if trying to bring the fingertips together and hold for a moment. Press firmly enough to move the skin over the skull instead of pulling her hair. Let go and rest your hands on her shoulders for a few moments.

What Next?

Now that you've tried out the techniques in this book, you should be able to give a relaxing or reviving massage – for friends as well as your lover. It will become more and more effective as you refine your skills and adapt to your partner's preferences.

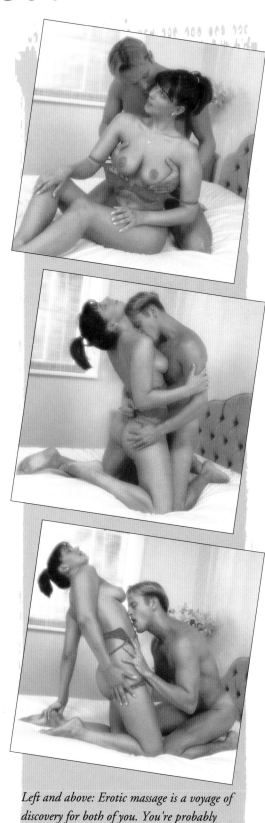

If the techniques in this book have inspired you to develop your skills further, look out for classes in your area. Massage is now so popular that there are training videos available for beginners, to rent or buy from good video outlets. And treat yourselves to a professional massage – as well as enjoying the treatment you could pick up some new ideas to try out at home.

Doctors, physiotherapists, holistic health centre staff and beauticians may be able to recommend reputable courses and practitioners. As with any holistic therapist, personal recommendation is useful so ask around among your friends. All these are, of course, for standard professional massage skills – the erotic element is one you add when practising with your lover.

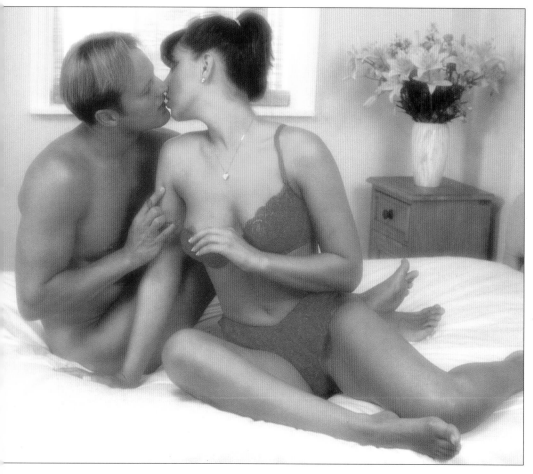

Left and above: Erotic massage is a voyage of discovery for both of you. You're probably discovering as much about your own body's capacity for sensual pleasure as about your lover's.

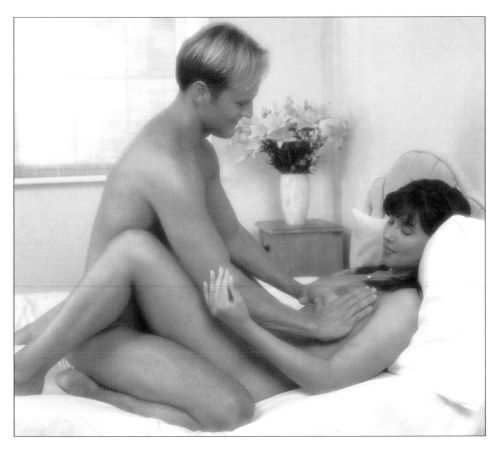

In adverts, people may call themselves a masseur or masseuse, the French words that tend to be used instead of the rather long-winded 'massage therapist'. Masseur (pronounced mass-*er*) simply means a man who gives massage and masseuse (pronounced mass-*erz*) is the female equivalent.

If you have stiff muscles – and most of us have – a therapeutic massage can be quite painful in the areas where we hold most tension – commonly in and just above the buttock muscles and across the shoulders. But the discomfort should not persist after the therapist stops touching the spot. Always mention in advance if you have any injuries or health conditions. And it's perfectly acceptable to ask a therapist to move on from a painful area or to press less hard – it's not meant to be an endurance test!

Left: Take time along the way to pause and simply enjoy the closeness you're sharing.

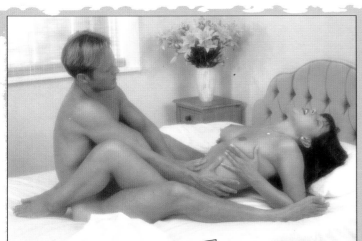

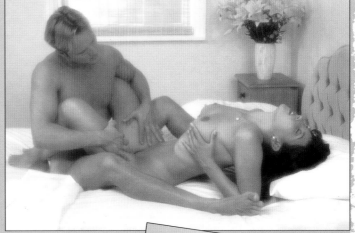

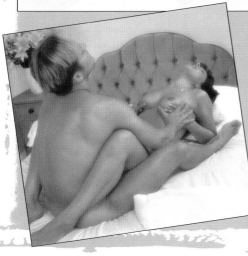

By this time you'll have learned a lot more about what feels good, how you most like being touched in different places and how your state of mind influences your enjoyment. To go further, why not treat yourselves to a professional massage, a video or even a short course. These will teach you more about the wide range of standard massage techniques, then you can discover their erotic potential when you're practising on each other.

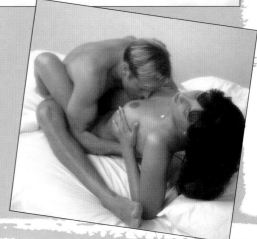

Index

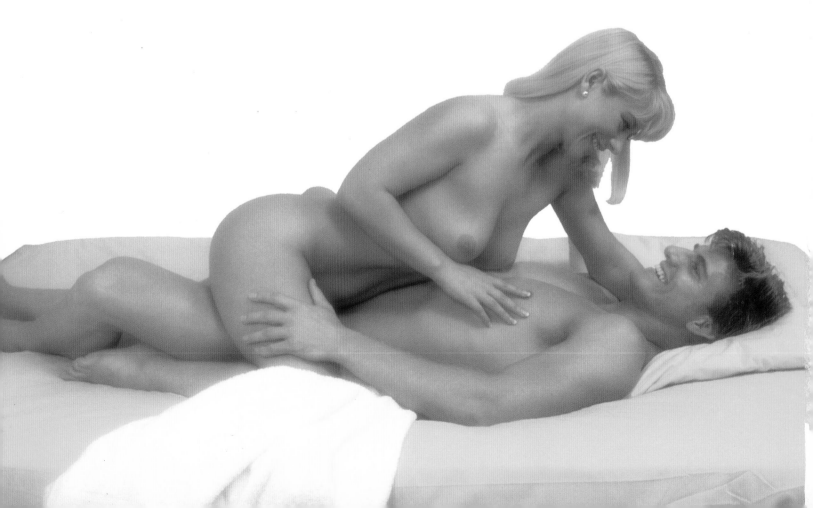